Grief Day By Day

Grief
DAY by DAY

Simple Practices and Daily Guidance
for Living with Loss

Jan Warner

ALTHEA
PRESS

To grief warriors around the world
and the people who love them.

To my beloved husband, Arthur Warner.
I love you. You're my heart. Always.

To my daughter, Erin, and my granddaughter, Gwendolyn,
who open my heart wider every day with fun and love.

To my friends all around the world
who love and accept me as I am.

Contents

Foreword

"Broken open" is the phrase I often use when grief wells up inside of me. Grief breaks one's heart wide open, and even though we work at healing that brokenness every day, we are always vulnerable to even the smallest occurrence that may shake it loose once more. Being in touch with those feelings is a reminder that the losses we've endured are profound.

Jan Warner's writing about her relationship with grief reaches into those cracks we try so hard to fill. With this book, Jan has created a beautiful ritual—an offering, really—that provides a connection for all of us, because "grief is our common language."

As I move through the themes and "exercises" in Jan's book, my tears are flowing once again, prompting me to notice how deeply my feelings fall, and how important it is to pause and hold those feelings for however long they need to rise and be.

There is nothing I can write here that Jan, coupled with the power of other writers' words, has not already artfully crafted. What I can share is my own relationship with loss and the inevitable jumble of feelings that follows. Everyone's experience with grief is uniquely their own, and Jan reminds us that grief is "messy."

As with many of our life experiences, what we carry from our parents and generations past seeps into our souls. My mother experienced devastating loss while she was pregnant with me. My family often reminded me that I cried for the first year and a half of my life and that my mother was the only one who could console me. I believe she and I shared a grief connection—my tears were the manifestation of her deep sorrow. I've always been a very sensitive and emotional person—perhaps that is why I pursued a career in acting. Even though the focus of my work has been in comedy, I was always able to tap into the pain that resides deep inside of me. I've walked through the loss of many relationships, including my brother Danny's death when we were both in our twenties. Jan suggests that death can deepen your relationship with God or a higher power; it certainly did for me when Danny died. He was close to God while he lived, and I had a knowingness that he was close to God in afterlife. His spirit has remained by my side throughout the decades, as has my mother's. Her death created a deep chasm in my heart, and much of my grieving for her has been in solitude, because my family dynamic shifted after her death. I still grieve the loss every day, but I am also able to find her in life's joyous moments, offering me peace.

Finding Jan's book now, finding her friendship and her ability to bring us to the core of the greatest tragedy of life—death—has given me great comfort. It's as if someone has extended a loving hand for me to hold as I continue my journey day by day.

—AMANDA BEARSE
Actor, Director, Producer & Teacher

Introduction

Take my hand and walk with me a while through the barren fields of grief. Is it true that this rocky soil, when watered with our tears, can still grow food to nourish our body and beautiful flowers to nourish our soul?

My husband, Artie, was charming, handsome, and stubborn. He lied to me about his age when I met him—I soon discovered he was 21 years older than I was. Imagination told me that his death would cause me great sadness and that I would miss him very much. When he died, I was so totally blown apart that when he didn't come back to get me, I thought it was my purpose to go to him. I didn't kill myself to make that journey only because I could not be the cause of others' grief.

Choosing life meant I needed to figure out how to be fully alive with grief. I started showing up at places where life was, in the hope that a bit of life would seep back into me. I went to a therapist. She told me I had "complicated grief," and that I should stop mourning my husband in six months to a year. She was a wonderful therapist, but I thought that was the most ridiculous thing I had ever heard. Why would I stop mourning a person who had been central to every part of my life? I didn't need to let go to move forward. I needed help in finding a home within myself for my grief.

I went to a bereavement group. I hadn't changed the bedsheets for three months. I met someone who hadn't changed their sheets for a year. I met someone else who had never changed them. I learned that I wasn't crazy; I was just grieving.

I thought all my grief work made me too sad, so I took a course in comedy sketch writing. When the teacher asked, "Why are you here?" I said, "My husband died so I thought I'd do comedy." I started storytelling. To my surprise, after my first storytelling show, people came up and thanked me for being honest about death and grief.

My husband was a recovering alcoholic who was always available to drunks and addicts. In an attempt to find meaning for my continued existence, I decided to make myself available to other grieving people as a way to honor my husband. I started a blog, "Stop Thief: Don't Steal My Grief," and a community on Facebook, Grief Speaks Out. I thought if I could reach one person, that would be enough. Grief Speaks Out now has more than 2.5 million likes from almost every country in the world. Grief is our common language.

Shortly after my husband died, I bought a sign that read, "Have an adequate day." It made me smile. I could have an adequate day even if I wasn't having a good day. I spent endless hours lying in bed. I had a rule that I could only stay in the house one day in a row, even if I only went out for five minutes on those other days. I assigned myself a "chore of the day" to give me a feeling of accomplishment, a chore as simple as paying one bill or just taking a shower. In addition to showing up for things whether I wanted to or not, I started helping people. Even from my bed, I could look online for others to connect to, who were also suffering, and I could post something supportive and encouraging. My husband used to say, "We only have moments." My goal was to have more happy and productive moments.

I traveled around the world experiencing various therapeutic modalities. I have a master's degree in counseling, but I realized I needed to try to save my own life. I'm an ordinary person. I still have times of utter collapse. I still have times, when wrestling with grief, that I find myself pinned down with no sense of myself or ability to move. Yet in the past eight years I have made many new friends. Some of them are fellow grievers. I have suffered, as many grievers have, the loss of dear friends who abandoned me or were unkind to me. Grief does that. I don't know why some people walk away when they are most needed, but they do.

I wanted so badly to die, but I would have missed so much. I did a one-woman show. I produced documentaries and an off-Broadway play. I started traveling again. When my daughter was pregnant, I honestly didn't know if I could love another human being. I can. Completely and with unexpected joy. My favorite role in life is being a grandmother. I still want to be with my husband in the same form, but I also want to have earthly adventures. It helps me to remember that what seems forever in earth years is a blink of an eye in terms of eternity.

Now I have written this book for you, for me, for us.

Take my hand and walk with me through these pages. Take what you need and leave the rest. As fellow grief warriors, let us find a way to celebrate through our own actions the lives of our loved ones, to make their lives matter more to us than their deaths.

How to Use This Book

This is your book and there is no right or wrong way to use it. You may start at week 1 and end at week 52, using one quote per day, in order. You may leaf through the book and start wherever you wish. You may reflect on one theme for a week or move around. You may return to one theme or quote many times. If something seems useful, use it. If something doesn't apply to you, move on to something else.

This book invites you to consider a different theme each week. There are 52 themes, one for each week of the year. Within each theme are quotes with a reflection for each day of the week. Each quote is meant to help you examine the theme from various perspectives. At the end of each week, you'll find a "Becoming a Grief Whisperer" exercise.

Why "Grief Whisperer"? A person who excels at calming or training difficult animals using gentle methods based on an understanding of the animal's natural instincts is often called a "whisperer," and there is no more difficult beast than grief. Understanding grief and finding you are not alone in your feelings as you use each exercise will help you train and thereby gentle-down your grief. The eventual goal, in your own time and in your own way, is to develop a relational home for your grief. I cannot promise that your grief will go away or even that you will want it to, but with time and practice you will learn to let grief inspire you rather than deaden you. You can begin to see the love that is reflected in grief. How do I know this? Many of these exercises have helped me as well as many other people. I still have dark and troubled times, but I now have skills I didn't have in the first chaotic year of grieving. I have learned to often feel fully alive with grief.

Again, choose the exercises that work for you. You can do them in order, or do whichever one you want. Do them one at a time, or do one or several over and over again. It may be helpful to keep a journal or a scrapbook to use with this book, to write things down, draw pictures, or include photographs or notes.

One word of caution: Sometimes it is helpful to do the one thing we absolutely do not want to do. Where we are most resistant can be where we are most stuck. If we can shake the stuck part loose, it allows other parts to begin to move.

You cannot do anything wrong. You are exactly where you are supposed to be. It is the nature of grief to be always shifting. You may feel you are doing fine, and then it all falls apart. This is normal. There is even a term for this: grief bursts, or grief attacks. Grief is not linear. There is no outward standard. People often write to me and ask if something is normal. I no longer ask myself that question. "Normal" is different for different people. Instead, I ask myself if something serves the kind of life I want to live. If it does, I accept it. If it doesn't, I see if I can change it. If I can't change it, I am patient with myself. I am grieving. Sometimes breathing is enough.

I often think of my grief as a sunflower. The center is always dark. My grief is dark and unchanging. Why shouldn't it be? I will always miss my husband. But the yellow petals surrounding the center are bright and numerous. At the beginning, my poor sunflower hardly had any petals. However, by nurturing it and allowing it to grow, the sunflower's dark center is now surrounded with many brightly colored petals; all the moments I have had since that impossible day in 2009 when my husband took his last breath.

I firmly believe that the depth of our grief measures the height of our love. I also believe that love triumphs over death, if we let it.

Stages of Grief?

Did you notice the question mark? The stages of grief, identified by psychiatrist Elisabeth Kübler-Ross, are often listed as denial, anger, bargaining, depression, and acceptance. I long suspected that even Elisabeth Kübler-Ross herself had not believed that these stages come in any orderly fashion, and that there is no time limit for passing through one, let alone all, of the stages. This suspicion was confirmed by grief expert David Kessler, who worked directly with her. So if anyone—even a professional— tells you that you are not grieving properly, don't take it to heart. Know that you are grieving exactly the way you are supposed to.

Day One

"The reality is that you will grieve forever. You will not 'get over' the loss of a loved one; you will learn to live with it. You will heal and you will rebuild yourself around the loss you have suffered. You will be whole again but you will never be the same. Nor should you be the same nor would you want to."

—ELISABETH KÜBLER-ROSS

Some people question her use of the word "heal," as well as the capacity of a grieving person to be whole again. To me, the important part is the simple statement that after a loss we will never be the same, and why would we want to? The quote acknowledges the duality of the griever: the ability to learn how to be fully alive while knowing that loss has changed us forever.

Day Two

"If you are working with a therapist . . . or anyone else who is trying to help you navigate the wilderness of grief and they start talking about the groundbreaking observations of Elisabeth Kübler-Ross suggesting there is an orderly predictable unfolding of grief please please please. Do yourself a favor. Leave . . . Grief is wild and messy and unpredictable."

—TOM ZUBA

It is unfortunate when those you seek out for help do not understand grief. In the name of helping, they want to label your grief process and show you the "inappropriateness" of certain feelings. You have the right to your own personal grief journey. Learning that the very nature of grief is to be surprising in its intensity and longevity is more useful than being given impractical goals to meet. If you are about to ride an untamed horse, isn't it better to be told that, rather than being told you are getting on a gentle pony?

Day Three

"Grief is not linear. People kept telling me that once this happened or that passed, everything would be better . . . But it is not linear . . . It is a jumble. It is hours that are all right, and weeks that aren't. Or it is good days and bad days. Or it is the weight of sadness making you look different to others and nothing helps."

—ANN HOOD

Grief takes a jumbled and disjointed path; one that is framed with both sadness and joy. It is in the darkest times we can learn to recall the glimmer of joy. In her blog Ann writes: "Oh! The human spirit never fails me. How we ache! How we love so deeply!"

Day Four

"[Some] psychologists out there will tell you that grief is a process . . . Others say that grief should only last two years at the most, otherwise it's 'abnormal' . . . Take away a person's grief and guaranteed they'll only be a frozen shell of a human being afterwards. Grief is only love, it's nothing to hide or send away with happy pills. Grief is a lifeline connecting two people who are in different realms together, and it's a sign of loyalty and hope."

—REBECCA MCNUTT

When I listen to the stories of grieving people, I try to focus on the love rather than the pain. The sadness that lasts for the rest of our lives is born out of the grace of this love. Grief remains a lifeline connecting us, and the loyalty and hope implied by this connection can show us how to find inspiration in our grief.

Day Five

"Grief, as I read somewhere once, is a lazy Susan. One day it is heavy and underwater, and the next day it spins and stops at loud and rageful, and the next day at wounded keening, and the next day numbness, silence."

—ANNE LAMOTT

With grief, as time goes by, we regain some control over what the lazy Susan offers us and how fast it spins. It may not be a steady control, but some control comes with what we learn day by day.

Day Six

"Apparently there were seven stages of grief but that was a neat way of putting it. Grief was messy and didn't [color] inside the lines."

—EMILY GALE

Whether you are a person who always colors inside the lines or a person who never colors inside the lines, you will likely be surprised at how messy grief is. It doesn't fit in boxes or stages and is not contained by lines. It goes where it wants and how it wants. Because of this, although taming grief is possible, it is not easy.

Day Seven

"The five stages—denial, anger, bargaining, depression, and acceptance—are a part of the framework that makes up our learning to live with the one we lost. They are tools to help us frame and identify what we may be feeling. But they are not stops on some linear timeline in grief."

—ELISABETH KÜBLER-ROSS

Here Kübler-Ross confirms that her five stages of grief are only tools to help us understand what we are feeling. They are not meant to be experienced once then never revisited. You might have anger mixed with depression. You might accept the death of the person you love most on Tuesday and refuse to accept it on Wednesday. You might think you have left bargaining behind, but then there it is again. You might have feelings and stages of your very own that are not on anyone else's list. You aren't crazy. You are grieving.

Becoming a Grief Whisperer

Write your own personal stages of grief. They can be descriptive of how you feel, have felt, and think you will feel in the future. They can be orderly or erupt all over the page. Or draw two maps: one is your actual grief journey; the other, what you would like your grief journey to be. What's your final destination—can you even imagine one? What are the places you need to visit along the way?

Loneliness

One of the most painful parts of grief is the loneliness. No matter how many people are in our lives, missing that one person makes the whole world seem empty. No one can replace those who have died. Even if we remarry, or have another child, or adopt another pet, no one will ever be the person loved in this specific way, in this specific time. This is why grief lasts, and in some ways loneliness, too, for the rest of our lives. Accepting this loneliness is part of who I am. It doesn't stop me from having good and strong loving relationships. I think of my loneliness for my husband as a way of keeping a space for him. It is a way of honoring the love we share.

Day One

"There's nothing lonelier than grief. Sometimes I wanted to cry out . . . 'Please please look at me help me can't you see how unhappy I am?' But . . . they would have gathered round making soothing noises . . . maybe offering me tissues . . . and none of that would touch the deep dark ocean that circled silently inside . . . "

—JOHN MARSDEN

This is the loneliness of grief. You want people to understand and pay attention to the part of you that is sad, that is in hiding, yet you know there is nothing they can do to help. The only thing that would really help is the impossible: to have your loved one come back. Does this loneliness ever go away? Yes and no. I spend more time in company now than I did when my husband first died. I have moments when I am busy and I forget how lonely I am—lonely for a specific person.

Day Two

> "There's grief and then there's the loneliness of grief. The way it's just yours and yours alone."
>
> —DEB CALETTI

While many other people also love and miss my husband, it doesn't make grief a shared activity. We each had a special treasured relationship with him, and although it's nice to hear stories about him and know he is remembered and loved and cried over, he is mine in a special way, as is my grief. It may sound a bit odd, but the specialness of our relationship makes the loneliness of my grief special, too. It took a long time, but there are now ways in which I am actually grateful for the loneliness of my grief.

Day Three

> "I miss your face. That big bright smile. You always had it, in any weather. It's hard for me to find one these days. These cold November days. Except when I think of you."
>
> —KELLIE ELMORE

I use this quote to illustrate loneliness because it tells me why I am lonely. What I miss is not any old smiling face. I miss one face in particular, one that no longer exists tangibly. Part of me cannot accept that the face I love so much does not exist except in memory and photographs. Loneliness for the physicality of my beloved sometimes makes it hard to smile. Thinking of him always makes me smile, even if the smile comes with tears or rage or fear or confusion.

Day Four

"It is true that the grief journey is very lonely, but it is also up to you to decide just how lonely you will make it."

—ELIZABETH BERRIEN

Is it truly possible to decide how lonely my grief journey is? May I have choice in how I experience grief? My loneliness feels deep and forever but perhaps I can say and do things that give me a different feeling. If I allow for the possibility of my loneliness lessening, a space for healing may open up. I can be lonely and not lonely at the same time.

Day Five

"No one ever has the answers you need, the ones you want most, the ones you whisper as you lay alone in your bed with the lights extinguished and the lonely ache of loss settling in."

—LEE THOMPSON

When someone we love dies, we have so many questions and no answers. Our world is shattered and we don't know how to put the pieces back together. Sometimes we don't even know if we want to. Nothing makes sense anymore. Some people feel that the lonely ache of loss increases rather than decreases over time. Yet that loneliness is because of love. The love illuminates the loneliness and in time can comfort it. Love is the glue that begins to mend the broken pieces.

Day Six

"Then I realized there was no one else to call, which was the saddest thing. The only person I really wanted to talk to about Augustus Water's death was Augustus Water."

—JOHN GREEN

Even after more than eight years, something will happen in my life and I go through the list of people in my mind I could call to share it with. It is a fairly long list, but most of the time I don't end up calling anyone because the only one I want to share it with is my husband. I want to talk about my husband's death with my husband. I want to hear his voice, see the look in his eyes, watch the corners of his mouth turn up in a smile. It's a quandary: The one person I shared everything with, still want to share everything with, is no longer alive.

Day Seven

"What no one told me about grief is how lonely it is. No matter who else is mourning, you're in your own little cell. Even when people try to comfort you, you're aware that now there is a barrier between you and them, made of the horrible thing that happened, that keeps you isolated."

—JODI PICOULT

I've heard many grieving people talk about how lonely they feel even in a crowd of people, as if we are not quite occupying the same space as everyone else. Can we reach through the barrier that grief has put between us and other people, between life and us? Will we ever feel present and alive in a way that shatters grief? Again, we live always in possibility. But there is no time limit for achieving this. There is also no failure in connecting one moment and returning to lonely isolation the next.

Becoming a Grief Whisperer

Close your eyes. Look into your loved one's remembered eyes. Put out your hand to feel their hand in yours. Breathe evenly and quietly if you can. Ask them to be with you for a while. Ask them if they have any advice for you on how to live without them still being alive with you. If you do not hear anything, imagine what they would say. Often imagination opens a door to communications.

Memory

Are my memories of my dead all that I have? No. I make new memories every day. However, I only have old memories with my husband. Will I allow grief to make my memories a source of sadness and pain, or will I reclaim them and let them bring me joy? I remember everything: the times we were very loving to each other, the times we fought, the times I felt lonely. I want to remember my husband as he was and remember us as we were. One way I keep my husband alive is by talking about him. Whether your loved one lived a long life or you bear the sadness of a miscarriage or a child born sleeping, you always have memories. Memory is a place I like to visit.

Day One

"Memories warm you up from the inside. But they also tear you apart."

—HARUKI MURAKAMI

Memories give us warmth and sustenance. Conversely, it is the feeling that they can never be repeated that tears us apart. Each season when roses bloom, I remember calling my husband to the back door. We held hands as we looked at the roses blooming in our garden. It is good when a memory brings warmth and, for a moment, doesn't tear us apart.

Day Two

"Memory, when it juts, retreats, recovers, shows us how to hold the darkness, how to breathe."

—DREW MYRON

My experience of grief was nothing I could have expected. The darkness was complete. In the beginning, I considered the possibility of light but I didn't see any way to get there. I didn't know that perhaps I was already there and didn't know it. I didn't even know how I could keep breathing, but I was breathing. Part of my becoming (in good moments) fully alive with grief was aided by the blessing of having so many memories of life and love with my husband. My memories, when I learned how to make them whole again, showed me how to hold the darkness and breathe.

Day Three

"Our memories of our loved ones are the pearl we form around the grain of grief that causes us pain."

—JEFF ZENTNER

Pearls are formed by substances a mollusk secretes to protect itself from an irritant that is trapped within itself. Grief is a powerful irritant that traps us and is trapped inside us. What if we can use our memories to protect us from this irritant? If grief is not going to go away, what if we can create something beautiful around it—with memory?

Day Four

"I was looking at the photographs and I started thinking that there was a time when these weren't memories."

—STEPHEN CHBOSKY

Photographs, like memories, can bring pleasure or pain or measures of both. The many photographs of my husband in my home are positioned where I have to choose to look at them. I love his face, but sometimes the fact that his face is no longer in the world fills me with sadness or anger. When those photographs were taken, I never thought they would be a large part of what I have left of him.

Day Five

"The archaeology of grief is not ordered. It is more like earth under a spade, turning up things you had forgotten. Surprising things come to light: not simply memories, but states of mind, emotions, older ways of seeing the world."

—HELEN MACDONALD

Some people are frightened they will forget their memories. That is part of my pleasure: I forget a memory and rediscover it. Did something really happen the way I remember it? It doesn't matter. In memories, I find feelings, I find opinions, and most importantly, I find love.

Day Six

"Why are the photographs of him as a little boy so incredibly hard to look at? Something is over. Now instead of those shiny moments being things we can share together in delighted memories, I, the survivor, have to bear them alone. All I can do is remember him, I cannot experience him. Nothing new can happen between us."

—NICHOLAS WOLTERSTORFF

I can remember, but we can no longer remember together. We can no longer argue about whose memory is accurate and whose isn't. We can no longer laugh and cry together. In some ways, for me the memory is even stronger, more precious. I am the keeper of my loved one's stories. I make the memory come alive. That is a responsibility that gives meaning to my life.

Day Seven

"What we have once enjoyed deeply we can never lose. All that we love deeply becomes a part of us."

—HELEN KELLER

It gives me comfort to think that while death has taken away my living husband, it cannot take away my enjoyment of the time we had together unless I let it. Those we love deeply become a part of us. While time can sometimes increase the hardship, it also increases my capacity for joy because of the ever-increasing ways I feel my husband being part of me. I love him more, not less. I feel him continuing to hold my hand and lead me forward. Is it that way for you?

Becoming a Grief Whisperer

One of the saddest, strongest weapons that grief has is its ability to taint our memories. This exercise, "Rolling your Memories Backward," helped me. Please modify anything that will help make this experience specific to you. It has been used with great success with soldiers with PTSD and with civilians.

Lie down or sit in a comfortable place. Play upbeat music if you wish. Choose a memory that has many aspects to it, a time filled with happiness as you experienced it. Roll it back in time. You are not thinking of the death of the person you love. You have no sense of the intensity of grief. When you feel that you are securely in the past, at the time the memory occurred, look around. What do you see, hear, touch, taste, smell, and physically feel? Be as specific as you can. What's the weather like? What is being said? What are the background noises? If the present enters, gently remind yourself that you are firmly in the past. Become conscious of your feelings. Do you feel warmth, safety, joy, or any other good feelings? Spend as much time deeply bathed in these good feelings as you like. When you are ready, knowing you can always return, wrap yourself in these good feelings. If you wish, place a "shield" around the memory or infuse it with white light.

Now, at a pace that is just right for you, return to the present, bringing the memory back with you. Let the memory be as it was when it happened. It's now firmly attached to all the good feelings that belong to it by its very nature.

Who Am I Now?

It is common to feel a sense of confusion about who you are when someone you love dies. This is because until they die, we don't necessarily realize how much our personality is tangled up with their personality. The pieces of your personality may seem broken and unfamiliar. You may feel as if you have also died. It is common to find that things you once loved now hold little enjoyment. However, bit by bit, you will find who you are. Will the person you are now ever feel like the old you? It might not. It might always feel a bit wobbly or different. That is okay.

Day One

"Even if you are alive somewhere, the absence of the other person who used to be there beside you obliterates your presence. Everything in the room, even the stars in the sky, can disappear in a second, changing one scene for another, just like in a dream."

—HWANG SOK-YONG

After my husband's death, I would say, "We died" when I meant to say, "He died." When he was alive, I did not realize how connected we were. We were independent people. I traveled all over the world by myself, as far as Timbuktu and back. No matter where I was or what I did, it was with the comfortable knowledge that he was at home waiting for me. His absence destroyed my feeling of presence, my feeling of being alive or wanting to be alive. It took me a long time to feel like a complete person again. I have created a new presence for him. It is not like the living, breathing him, but it helps me to live.

Day Two

"Who in the world am I? Ah, that's the great puzzle."

—LEWIS CARROLL (CHARLES DODGSON)

Figuring out who you are when your loved one is no longer alive is a puzzle that takes creativity, time, and courage. It's a puzzle that may fall to pieces again and again. Over time, the puzzle will fit together again, but it will be a different shape than you have ever known. You have within you the possibility of being an amazing person, but you will never be the same person you were.

Day Three

"The obliterated place is equal parts destruction and creation. The obliterated place is pitch black and bright light. It is water and parched earth. It is mud and it is manna. The real work of deep grief is making a home there."

—CHERYL STRAYED

It can be easier to be blinded by the "obliterated place," making the creation part hard to find. We see the pitch black and can't find the bright light. We see the cracked, parched earth, and water is nowhere to be found. All mud, no manna. But when you are ready, you may notice how creative you are, how much light you carry within you. Every griever carries the bright light of love. That is grief work, making a home and finding a home in grief.

Day Four

"I'm afraid it won't stop, and all my bones will disappear and one day I'll just dissolve. I won't be able to stand up anymore, or move. Mostly I'm afraid that it won't matter. Because I have nowhere to go, and nothing to do . . . There isn't just a wound. There is a great gaping black hole that sucks all the light, all that mattered, into it."

—LOUISE PENNY

I, too, have felt that I no longer existed. I have felt that my physical as well as my emotional and spiritual being went off with my husband when he took his last breath. Then, like a magic trick, one that I didn't even know I was performing, parts of me began to take form. I showed up places where life was and waited for it to seep back into me. I helped other people and in doing so, helped myself. After eight years I am here. If I disappear, I can come back in an hour or day instead of after huge swaths of lost time. I am a grieving, off-balance person, but I am a person. I suppose I always was. If we look at ourselves through our loved one's loving eyes instead of our own, we see ourselves differently. We can let their belief in us replace our self-doubt.

Day Five

"If you were to find a shattered mirror, find all the pieces . . . and have whatever skill and patience it took to put all that broken glass back together . . . the restored mirror would still be spiderwebbed with cracks, it would still be a useless glued version of its former self, which could show only fragmented reflections of anyone looking into it."

—ELIZABETH WURTZEL

The death of someone central to our life can make our very being feel shattered. In attempting to piece the broken shards back together, we may find we do not know who we are anymore. But something unexpected can happen. Within this discomfort, we can be surprised by finding new strengths, new attributes that we hadn't known before our great sadness.

Day Six

"The dead aren't the only ones who vanish: you, too, can disappear in plain sight if enough is taken from you. I was still missing, in many ways. And I wasn't sure I wanted to be found."

—SARAH DESSEN

Do I want to find myself or be found by others? I don't want to be alone and I don't want to be with others. It's easy to isolate and necessary to be part of the world. To keep myself to this, my first rule is to show up. My calendar contains both plans with others and resting places. If people choose isolation, I have empathy, not judgment. But, for me, making sure I don't vanish means being seen by others. The moments I don't want to be found are often the times when I most need to find myself and let others find me as well.

Day Seven

"Nobody can teach me who I am. You can describe parts of me, but who I am—and what I need—is something I have to find out myself."

—CHINUA ACHEBE

It is a rare person who can connect enough to teach me something that helps me discover who I am again; many waste words by offering useless platitudes. I need what I can't have—I need my dead to come back. If you miss that essential piece, you miss the center of who I am. Someone once asked, "How are you?" I answered, "Fine, thank you. Of course, my husband is still dead." The people who are most helpful never tell me who I am or how I should act or feel. Instead, they show me ways to discover new things about myself. And people who share their own experiences make me feel less alone and able to see other paths to take.

Becoming a Grief Whisperer

This exercise helps us get in touch with ever increasing aspects of ourselves.

You can practice this exercise out loud or in writing, by yourself or with a partner.

Fill in the following blanks: I am _____. Yes, I am _____, but I am also _____. (You can also use I feel _____ instead of I am _____, then Yes, I feel _____, but I also feel _____.)

For example: "I am a griever. Yes, I am a griever, but I am also a writer. I am a writer, but I am also a helper. Yes, I am a helper, but I am also someone who stays in bed too much. Yes, I am someone who stays in bed too much, but I am also someone who likes to take walks. I feel sad all the time. Yes, I feel sad all the time, but I also feel happy when I see pictures of puppies. Yes, I feel happy when I see pictures of puppies, but I also get angry a lot. Yes, I get angry a lot, but I also enjoy playing Scrabble. You can use it in a sentence. I am stuck. Yes, I am stuck, but I am someone who keeps going."

Repeat your sentences a minimum of 25 times. It is important to continue to do more reflecting and repeating when you are feeling most stuck.

Beauty

One of the vicious things that grief does is rob us of the ability to see and appreciate beauty. Beauty and color are gone; it is a black-and-white world empty of delight. If we do find something to delight in, we might feel guilty. Grief work is finding things and places in the world to give our grief a cushion to rest on. Beauty is there; beauty is everywhere. Stretch out your hand to hold your loved one's hand. Let them help you open your eyes again. Let them help you find beautiful things reappearing everywhere.

Day One

"I've found that there is always some beauty left—in nature, sunshine, freedom, in yourself; these can all help you."

—ANNE FRANK

If a 13-year-old girl who knew of the terrors being perpetrated by the Nazis could find beauty, isn't it possible for us to do so, too, even in the midst of grief? Anne Frank found beauty in nature, sunshine, and freedom, and she found it helpful. Where can you find beauty? If you cannot see it yet, can you try?

Day Two

"Those who contemplate the beauty of the earth find reserves of strength that will endure as long as life lasts. There is something infinitely healing in the repeated refrains of nature—the assurance that dawn comes after night, and spring after winter."

—RACHEL CARSON

Grief can seem like an endless night, an endless winter. By contemplating the beauty of the earth and her rhythms, we remind ourselves that no matter how long the night, the sun always rises. There is suffering to be acknowledged, and there are things even greater than suffering that we learn once again to see. The earth is wide and big and the universe even more so. If we are too fragile to hold the enormity of our grief, we can share it with nature. The beauty and healing that exists outside can begin to permeate our hearts, our souls, our daily lives.

Day Three

"And when all the wars are over, a butterfly will still be beautiful."

—RUSKIN BOND

Is there a peace that can be declared in the battle with grief? I don't know, but I do know that butterflies are still beautiful. If we can look out of the window of our houses of grief and see the beauty in a butterfly, we have connected for a moment to something other. It is a sadness not to be able to share it with the person we most want to share it with, yet if we acknowledge it still exists, we can fly on its wings for a bit.

Day Four

"And that is just the point . . . how the world, moist and beautiful, calls to each of us to make a new and serious response. That's the big question, the one the world throws at you every morning. 'Here you are, alive. Would you like to make a comment?'"

—MARY OLIVER

Each minute of each day is a call to respond, to comment, to be. Each minute of each day we have a choice: to continue to sleep or arise, even for a moment; to keep the blindfold of grief secure or take it off and open our eyes again. As much as I want to be dead or feel dead, here I am, alive. The question remains, "What am I going to do with my life?" When will I be ready to answer with a resounding "yes" instead of with silence?

Day Five

"Many eyes go through the meadow, but few see the flowers in it."

—RALPH WALDO EMERSON

The meadow represents life, a huge canvas that cannot be looked at in its entirety. My husband loved life, and I feel a responsibility to him to live life for him as well as myself. I want eyes that will always look for and often see the flowers in the meadow. It helps me look with love. Grief is always a reminder of love.

Day Six

"You cry for a long time, and then after that are defeated and flattened for a long time. Then somehow life starts up again . . . Some aching beauty comes with huge loss, although maybe not right away when it would be helpful."

—ANNE LAMOTT

The problem is that we cannot often see the beauty through our grief. Grief can blot out even the sun. Perhaps as a child, you used a rainbow of crayons to draw a picture, then covered it all with black crayon. After, you scratched away at the black to reveal the color. Grief can be like that, and grief work involves this process of scratching away. This work is less about finding beauty and more about being willing to develop the ability to see it again. Grievers need spectacles for damaged eyes that allow beauty to be seen.

Day Seven

"As I got closer to it, it got brighter and brighter. It wasn't like any light I could describe to you. It was beautiful."

—JAMES L. GARLOW

We want our beloved dead to be somewhere beautiful. I imagine they want us to be somewhere beautiful as well. Earth seems a strange and lonesome place when the person we love most has died. Yet there is still great beauty here for us to enjoy until it is our time to see the beauty there.

Becoming a Grief Whisperer

At various times during your day, close your eyes. Open them. What do you see that is beautiful? In any environment, can you find at least one beautiful thing? You can simply notice and remember each thing, or you can write them down, draw them, or describe them into a recording device. By doing this, you're training yourself to see beauty again. If seeing beautiful things makes you sad or angry, see the exercise in week 3 (page 15). Remember what it was like to share beautiful things with your loved one. Bring those feelings with you into the present. Share the beauty with them in the present. Being fully alive with grief involves training ourselves to look in new places to find new things. We don't need to let go of sadness to let other emotions peek through and startle us with renewed wonder.

WEEK 6
Time

We have learned to measure time, yet when we're grieving, time loses all measure. For us, the world has stopped while others seem to quite rudely go on with their day. Grief is not anchored in the past. The trauma of grief occurs over and over again every day. Our loved ones don't die once. They die every second we think of them and know we have to live our life without them. Time goes by slowly and too fast. We cannot go back in time and make our loved ones alive again. How do we move forward and let love make our grief something that inspires us?

Day One

"Grief is forever. It doesn't go away; it becomes a part of you, step for step, breath for breath. I never stop grieving her because I never stop loving her. That's just how it is . . . All I can do is love her, and love the world, emulate her by living with daring and spirit and joy."

—JANDY NELSON

Time is now infused with grief. Every moment contains the knowledge of someone we love who has died. Every moment contains both love and pain. There is a challenge in this. My husband loved life. In what ways can we look at our loved one's life and emulate it? I have learned, in time, to take on some of my husband's energy and spirit. I go forward with his love inside me and radiating from me.

Day Two

"There are people whose death leaves you with an ache of grief. A slight sting. And then there are people whose death stops time. Deaths that leave the sky murky all day long because even the sun is grieving. Deaths that shut down your muscles and stop the music."

—PATRICIA AMARO

People don't always distinguish between the different kinds of grief. They may know someone who died and it didn't affect them very much, so they don't understand why other people are shattered by grief. Some people's deaths stop time. The world continues, but the griever stands still.

Day Three

"It has been said, 'time heals all wounds.' I do not agree. The wounds remain. In time, the mind, protecting its sanity, covers them with scar tissue and the pain lessens. But it is never gone."

—ROSE FITZGERALD KENNEDY

When we are grieving, people try to comfort us by suggesting that time heals. Time can lessen or change the nature of our pain. Each person's path is different, but all paths deal with the fact that we learn to hold the pain while we begin to live fully again. We are wounded, but we are still alive.

Day Four

"Time does not bring relief; you all have lied Who told me time would ease me of my pain!"

—EDNA ST. VINCENT MILLAY

The memory of our loved ones follows us everywhere. My husband never saw where I live now. It doesn't matter; each room is filled with his memory. We miss our loved ones every day, every place. Time does not change this. The change comes not with time passing, but with our learning to embrace what time gives us.

Day Five

"Grief resets the clock of life to before and after."

—LYNDA CHELDELIN FELL

Time runs differently for grieving people. Some people call it the new normal. Some people call it the new abnormal. There is life before the death of someone central to our existence, and life after. The through line between the two lives is love.

Day Six

"Grief is love turned into an eternal missing . . . It can't be contained in hours or days or minutes."

—ROSAMUND LUPTON

Missing someone is a continuing theme and a big part of a griever's life. It is bigger than time. There's no containing it. How does one become fully alive again while incorporating this sense of missing? Can missing turn from a dull ache or a sharp pain into a way to honor our loved one's memory? Can I become bigger than time? Can I become someone who cannot be contained?

Day Seven

"In the support group, the counselor had said: When you lose a loved one, you feel as if you're inside a confined space. Everyone else will seem to be careening along outside of this space. In time, you will become aware of an opening you are going to have to step through . . . You will step through."

—JAMIE QUATRO

When you're behind glass, watching the rest of the world go forward with their lives and maybe hating them for it, how do you choose to step through and rejoin them? I step through, but I also step back. It helps me to know I can step back. The solution for me, when I was ready, was not to try to keep up. I allow myself downtime to regain my strength.

Becoming a Grief Whisperer

Time travel. Close your eyes. If you like, play music softly. If it is helpful, set an alarm. Imagine what your time-travel machine looks like. What do the controls look like? Your time machine must be able to stop anywhere in the past, present, or future. It must be able to move slowly or quickly. It must automatically bring you back to the present time and place, but the you that comes back may have changed in some slight or significant way.

Decide where you want to go. Do you want to relive a specific memory? Go to a certain time in history? Perhaps there was something you were planning to do with your loved one. Once you've chosen a destination, decide how quickly you want to move. Adjust your controls, remembering to set the return dial to your present time and place.

When you arrive at your destination, spend as much time there as you like. Notice everything. When you are ready to return to the present, make a little package to bring back with you. It can be a memento, a souvenir, or simply a good feeling. Only bring with you something that will be of use or comfort. Also make a little package of something you want to leave behind, something you do not want with you in the present. Use your time travel machine as often as you want. Take it with you everywhere you go.

Fear

There is more than one kind of fear associated with grief. There is fear attached to real circumstances. Sometimes we depended on the person who died for practical things. Who will take care of me if I am ill? Free-floating anxiety is fear that is not attached to any particular thing. Life is frightening without our loved ones. I am perfectly safe, but this knowledge is not enough. My husband was my buffer, my safe place. There is also the fear that other people we love will die. The ground is no longer securely beneath our feet. Sometimes this fear is easily managed, but sometimes the death of someone we love can lead to PTSD and/or panic attacks. If this has happened to you, you are not alone.

Day One

"No one ever told me that grief felt so like fear."

—C.S. LEWIS

People tell you that the emotion associated with grief is sadness. Most cultures don't give us any preparation for grief. It feels like fear because certainty and trust have disappeared. The life you planned on, the life you took for granted is gone. Even when a death is expected, when it happens it is always a great fearful shock to our emotional, physical, and spiritual systems.

Day Two

"I keep finding myself stifled by the company of others and then crippled by loneliness when I leave them. I am terrified and I don't even know of what, because I have lost everything already."

—VERONICA ROTH

When one person has died, the whole world feels empty. It is normal to not want to be alone and not want to be with others. Both are frightening and uncomfortable. We don't feel we have lost a singular thing; we feel we have lost everything. Fear is a natural response.

Day Three

"I used to be afraid that if I experienced grief it would overcome me and I wouldn't be able to survive the flood of it, that if I actually felt it I wouldn't be able to get back up. It's taught me that I can feel it and it won't swallow me whole."

—ELISABETH KÜBLER-ROSS

I have often heard grief described as a black hole. Many of us fear that grief will consume us for the rest of our days, that it has delivered a knock-out punch from which there is no recovery. What we learn in time is that while the grief may remain, we can learn tools to tame it. Real strength is in being vulnerable: we can feel grief and joy.

Day Four

"Grief is terror, in its most undiluted form."

—MATT HAIG

Grief is not simply fear; it is terror. Terror of the unknown. Terror of living without those we love. This terror comes whether we have miscarried a wanted, loved child or been with someone their entire life. The terror comes in waves as you learn to bear the unbearable, endure the unendurable.

Day Five

"Death is such a tragic and scary thing. The grim reaper kidnapping our loved ones like a murderer and the living are left in a grief stricken panic. The griever now lives life like a wounded soldier with a hole in his heart and a hundred pound bag of sorrow strapped to his back."

—SUSIE NEWMAN

How often do people say our loved ones are "in a better place?" Perhaps they are. We're not. My heart is broken and I carry grief with me everywhere. Some people have panic attacks. Some people feel that everything has become more difficult, perhaps impossibly difficult. Grief work is carrying this load and feeling it lighten. It's having a heart beat with a hole in it, and learning how to be fully alive with grief.

Day Six

"What I was afraid of was my own grief . . . and the stark awareness I had of being, for the first time in my life, entirely alone, a Crusoe shipwrecked and stranded in the limitless wastes of a boundless and indifferent ocean."

—JOHN BANVILLE

Grief is indeed a feeling of being shipwrecked. It calls us to use tools we don't know we have. How will we survive? How will we become someone who doesn't merely survive, but thrive?

Day Seven

"Grief, our ally and companion, reminds us of a central truth that is hidden within our tears and fears: The one whom we grieve loved us. We are lovable."

—LISA IRISH

Here is the twist, a path through fear: Love. People who do not love, who are not loved, are spared grief. The path through all emotions associated with grief is love.

Becoming a Grief Whisperer

Find a comfortable place. Put on soothing music if you wish. Close your eyes. Think of a time or place when you felt safe. It can be real or imaginary. Use all of your senses to fill in even the tiniest detail. Choose if you wish to be there alone or invite people in. I always ask my husband to join me, a young, healthy version of himself. It doesn't matter where you go or what you do there. This is a place fear cannot enter. If you start to feel afraid in this place, arm yourself with a feather or sage or noisemaker—these are called anchors and will help you banish the fear. Become familiar with this place. Know that you can return whenever you choose.

When you return to the present, bring those feelings of comfort with you. If you used something to banish fear, see if you can find something similar. In real time, shake your noisemaker. Touch your feather. Burn a candle. Say a phrase if you desire. This might work the first time. It might be working but you don't notice it yet. It might work the second or third or fifth time. Fear may appear to teach you something and then vanish. Acknowledging what your fear is saying gives it permission to go away.

Confusion (Fog)

When my husband first died, I used to put my clothes on backward. I would look at the tags, adjust them, and put them on backward. I would take them off and adjust them, but they would still be on backward. This happens to me even now around certain dates. Some people call this confusion "grief brain." The only thing you don't need to be confused about is that your foggy brain is a normal reaction to grief.

Day One

> "For a long time I spent my weary days in a fog of what might be and what has been and I guess you could say I'm still learning how to accept what is."

—NIKKI ROWE

How do I accept what is? I spend time in the past. I spend time in a future that doesn't exist. Sometimes I am present, but often my present is overshadowed by swirling thoughts and feelings that leave me confused. This confusion can make even simple tasks difficult. This happens to many grievers as we learn to grieve with clarity as well as confusion.

Day Two

"I suppose that the human mind can only stand so much grief and anguish. After that the fuses blow."

—FYNN

The lights in my brain have gone out. The best I can do is know where the fuse box is. I can turn the lights back on and the confusion disappears. Then the fuses blow again, and again I have to fix them. The odd thing is how well we learn to live with this.

Day Three

"It hurts when they're gone. And it doesn't matter if it's slow or fast . . . When they're gone the world turns upside down and you're left holding on, trying not to fall off."

—WALTER MOSLEY

I used to wonder why people said they were surprised when someone who was elderly or had a terminal illness died. Now I know. You don't expect someone to die that day, that moment. Grief is often so much more intense and debilitating than we imagined it would be. While grieving, we learn to live in a confusing, upside-down world. We learn to hold on. We can even learn to laugh and enjoy life in the midst of it all.

Day Four

"Then there's the kind of zombie I've become now: the one who has lost everything—his brain, his heart, his light, his direction. He wanders the world, bumping into this, tripping over that, but keeps going and going. That is life after death."

—ADAM SILVERA

We are zombie grievers. We have lost everything. We live in confusion. We live in pain. But we keep going. How will we make this need to keep going into something useful, even delightful? When we are ready, we'll know.

Day Five

"Caught baffled by the perplexing slow-release of sadness for ever and ever and ever."

—MAX PORTER

We live with sadness, and it confuses everyday things. We find joy, but still the sadness continues. That's the life of a grief warrior, letting the river of sadness be merely a part of our landscape. Learning in time to build bridges over it, to use sandbags so it won't overflow its banks.

Day Six

"Grief is baffling . . . Some believe the range of
emotions mourners experience is predictable . . .
as if mourners are following a checklist. But sorrow
is less of a checklist, more like water. It's fluid, it has
no set shape, never disappears, never ends . . . It just
changes. It changes us."

—MIRA PTACIN

How can we sustain all the emotions tangled up with our grieving? No one
tells us how baffling it all is. Too often when we ask for help, we are told to
"suck it up, buttercup," and move on. This is not helpful. We are changed.
However flexible we are, we cannot learn something new without practice
and support.

Day Seven

"And as the ax bites into the wood, be comforted in the
fact that the ache in your heart and the confusion in
your soul means that you are still alive, still human,
and still open to the beauty of the world."

—PAUL HARDING

At first, I hated the fact I was still alive. I didn't want to be open to the
beauty of the world if I couldn't share it. In time I have learned to be fully
alive with grief because I want my husband to be proud of me. I want to
help people. I want to see beauty again because I am still sharing it with
him, only in a different way. The confusion in my soul is still there, but
whereas in the beginning I only had questions, now I have some answers.

Becoming a Grief Whisperer

Buy yourself activity books for children or adults that contain mazes. I recommend that you start with the children's ones to make this exercise easy and fun (if you're ready for fun). Along with the books, purchase some brightly colored markers, pens, or pencils. Each day, do as many mazes as you wish. Each time you complete a maze, you are training your brain to follow a path simply and clearly without confusion. Just as you complete a maze without confusion, you will, without even thinking about it, learn to navigate a task or social situation without confusion. If you find yourself stepping into confusion for a while, you now know you can also step out.

WEEK 9
Denial

Denial is a coping mechanism. It can be a friend or an enemy. I like pretending that my husband isn't dead. When he first died, I would come home and say, "Hi honey. Are you home? Oh, I must have missed you. I'll see you later." I want to be conscious of denial and how I am using it. If I actually sat and waited for my husband to come home, I would be in trouble—that denial is too deep. Sometimes there is a sense of humor in my denial. I use it to give my grief a place to rest for a while.

Day One

"It's not denial. I'm just selective about the reality I accept."

—BILL WATTERSON

Imagine a denial so deep that you are in denial about your denial! Active denial is a willingness to bend reality. If I hold my hand out and feel my loved one holding it, I know that is not actual reality. It is my reality but not objective reality. However, there are times when being selective about the reality we accept hurts no one. It can even be helpful.

Day Two

"Again, I stuffed down the grief and opened the door wide to denial. I may have looked okay on the outside, but inside I was an ugly hot mess."

—BETTS KEATING

Sometimes denial is necessary to survival. Wearing a mask and always pretending to be okay when you are falling apart inside is socially acceptable, but it can be corrosive. When you ask me how I am, I tend to tell you. However, I understand that for many grievers, silence is easier and therefore preferable.

Day Three

"If you asked me, denial was the best stage of grief. If prompted, the Wicked Queen's mirror would definitely say it was the fairest of them all."

—LAUREL ULEN CURTIS

I remember a dream I had in the beginning. I turned over in bed and saw my husband. I said, "Oh my God. I thought you were dead. I thought cancer killed you." He said, "Come here, you silly girl. Of course I'm not dead. What a nightmare!" Then I rolled over and curled up into his arms. That was the best denial I ever experienced. Definitely the fairest of them all. But then I woke up. That is what happens with denial. We wake up. What do we do then?

Day Four

"I am taking this in, slowly,
  Taking it into my body.
  This grief. How slow
  The body is to realize
  You are never coming back."

—DONNA MASINI

How many of us can't quite accept that someone we love so much is never coming back? Even years later, we think we see our loved ones in a crowd, or hear their voice. There is a big gap between our brain and our heart.

Day Five

"It's always been hard for me to tell the difference between denial and what used to be known as hope."

—MICHAEL CHABON

Denial is false hope. Real hope comes from feeling the depth of all emotions and having the courage to see a way through. It is sometimes as difficult as finding something to hold on to in a pit of quicksand, or as easy as finding a million stars in the darkest night.

Day Six

"Denial is as brittle as glass. It's solid until a force you never saw coming crashes into it and shatters the thin wall you've constructed to protect yourself from the truth."

—CANDACE KNOEBEL

This is something to prepare for: the aftershock when denial shatters. It is why sometimes in the middle of a happy moment we may burst into tears. How will I handle it when the great force of my grief hits me when I least expect it? As time has passed, this usually happens when I am alone rather than at the most uncomfortable times.

Day Seven

"It would mean . . . that those things that are meant for me as much as for anybody else—the beauty of the sun and moon, the pageant of the seasons, the music of daybreak and the silence of great nights . . . would all be tainted for me, and lose their healing power, and their power of communicating joy. To regret one's own experiences is to arrest one's own development . . . It is no less than a denial of the soul."

—OSCAR WILDE

May there come a time for you when denial of all reality has served its purpose, and like a flower's bud, you allow yourself to open again. May there come a time when the love you have and have been given allows your reality of the harsh and splendid world to no longer be tainted by grief. Let your grief be full of holes for joy, healing, and wonder to flow through.

Becoming a Grief Whisperer

Imagine a bowl. Your bowl can be any shape and size, and made out of anything you wish. When you see what your bowl looks like, take your two hands and hold your bowl just under your heart. Let all those emotions you have been denying because you are afraid of them or because they are too painful flow into your bowl. You do not need to name the emotions. You don't even have to feel them. Just let them flow out of you into your bowl. They can be any temperature, any consistency that they need to be. When your bowl is full, or even overflowing, tip it over and let the contents spill into the earth, which can absorb them without harm. Repeat this process as many times as you like. Take your bowl with you and do this exercise any time or place you wish. You will know when you feel the relief that comes from this cleansing.

Music

In the 1700s, Philip V of Spain, who suffered from severe depression, had the opera singer Farinelli leave the stage and become his personal singer, bringing him back to emotional health. Music has been used as a therapeutic tool for centuries and is uniquely effective in the treatment of physical and mental issues including depression, anxiety, and hypertension. While we cannot afford to hire our own singer as Philip V did, we do have access to music through many avenues. Through experimentation, we can discover which types of music are our personal grief healers. We can greatly benefit by incorporating music into our daily lives.

Day One

"Somewhere out in the darkness, a phoenix was singing in a way Harry had never heard before: a stricken lament of terrible beauty. And Harry felt . . . his own grief turned magically to song."

—J.K. ROWLING

Mythically, a phoenix is a bird that rises from ashes. Our task is to rise from the ashes of our grief. Is my grief something that I can turn into song? Will my grief always be a sad song, or can it be also a song of love and joy?

Day Two

"Music is a rainbow that captures our sorrows."

—TARESSA KLAYS

My grief often seems opaquely black. What if it becomes instead a cloak of many colors? What if tears refract light to make a rainbow? What color is your grief? What color can your grief become?

Day Three

"Then I played the song that hides in the center of me. That wordless music that moves through the secret places in my heart. I played it carefully, strumming it slow and low into the dark stillness of the night. I would like to say it is a happy song . . . sweet and bright, but it is not."

—PATRICK ROTHFUSS

What are the songs that hide in the center of you? Are they sad songs? It may be only the sad songs that you can hear and the joyous songs that you have to listen for. Can you begin to hear them? Are you ready?

Day Four

"It was a haunting tune, unresigned, a cry of heartache for all in the world that fell apart. As ash rose black against the brilliant sky, Fire's fiddle cried out for the dead, and for the living who stay behind and say goodbye."

—KRISTIN CASHORE

What music would there be that could echo the pain of the living who are left behind when those they love die? A music so expressive that all grievers feel their sorrow not only understood and expressed, but also elevated into something beyond words.

Day Five

"Music speaks what cannot be expressed. It soothes the mind and gives it rest. It heals the heart and makes it whole. It flows from heaven to heal the soul."

—K.C. LYNN

If music flows from heaven, does it come from our loved ones? Are they still singing to us while we dance? If we feel as though nothing can ever soothe our minds or heal our hearts, we can close our eyes and let the music's gentleness enter every cell of our body. Perhaps being repaired at this deep cellular level is something that is already happening. It will only be a matter of time until our consciousness becomes aware of it.

Day Six

"The ocean has been singing to me, and the song is that of our life together."

—NICHOLAS SPARKS

The song of our life together is where healing comes from. We have been given what so many long for. We have been given love. It might not be heaven, the ocean, or even nature that sings to you. Where does your music come from? What is it that gives you perhaps a brief glimpse of peace?

Day Seven

"Music was my refuge. I could crawl into the space between the notes and curl my back to loneliness."

—MAYA ANGELOU

Music presents us with a place to crawl into and be comforted. Can you find the space between the notes and, even if for just a brief moment and then perhaps a longer one, curl your back to loneliness? Feel your loved one curled up there beside you.

Becoming a Grief Whisperer

Spend time every day for at least a week exploring music and your relationship to it. "Solitude" by Louis Armstrong breaks my heart open. You may choose music that exposes your deeper feelings about your beloved dead, or music that allows you to escape into a grief-free world. Any type of music will do. Notice your response. You can do this sitting or lying down, or even dancing. If you wish, imagine your loved one dancing with you. You can sing, or write a song for your beloved. This is a free-form exercise that will allow you to deepen your relationship with music.

WEEK 11
Unhealthy Coping Mechanisms

I asked my good friend why, when we are stressed, we do the very things that make us weaker rather than stronger. It would be more sensible for me to take care of myself in ways that would strengthen my being. I know that exercising increases endorphins and can make my mood lighten. I know that eating healthy and not using substances can give me greater energy. It is not a matter of what I know; it is a matter of how I act. It is unfortunately common for a grieving person to try to blunt the pain of grief in unhealthy, even dangerous ways.

Day One

"**I have absolutely no pleasure in the stimulants in which I sometimes so madly indulge. It has not been in the pursuit of pleasure that I have periled life and reputation and reason. It has been the desperate attempt to escape from torturing memories, from a sense of insupportable loneliness and a dread of some strange impending doom.**"

—EDGAR ALLAN POE

Sometimes the pain of grief leads us to take various substances to escape. We have not yet learned to allow our memories to contain the joy they once did. We have not found anything to soften our loneliness. Grief is not depression or anxiety, although it can cause depression, anxiety, and other mental health concerns. There is a difference between responsibly taking medication prescribed by a doctor and trying to self-medicate. In a time of mental chaos, it can be difficult to make an informed decision. It is not always easy to look into our own heart and decide whether we need to seek help.

Day Two

"She lost much of her appetite. At night, an invisible hand kept shaking her awake every few hours. Grief was physiological, a disturbance of the blood . . . "

—JEFFREY EUGENIDES

After my husband died, I hardly ate at all. Grief made my stomach ache. Food didn't seem like nourishment. The brutal fact of our loved one's death might fade for a minute, but when it returns, it can leave us listless and unwilling to sustain even the motion of taking a bite of food. It is the life force within us, and our loved ones—the living and the dead—that encourage us to take care of ourselves.

Day Three

"In Louisiana, one of the first stages of grief is eating your weight in Popeye's fried chicken. The second stage is doing the same with boudin. People have been known to swap the order. Or to do both at the same time."

—KEN WHEATON

I soon returned to my compulsive need to use food as comfort rather than nourishment. If sugar was illegal, like heroin and cocaine, I might find myself in a prison cell. I'm not sure why eating too much seems like a solution to grief. Overeating is not for the joy of food—it's immediate gratification to distract from pain, to create numbness. Addiction feels like self-care, but it is the opposite, and it can be deadly as well as deadening.

Day Four

"I took a drink, wiping my mouth with the back of my hand, repeating the gesture that was made a hundred times by my father and his father and his father's father, eyes half closed as the sharpness of the alcohol replaced the sharpness of grief."

—NICOLE KRAUSS

My husband was a recovering alcoholic. He said he was one of the miracles. Alcohol can warm the body and the soul and give the illusion that we are functioning human beings as we continue to unravel. A drink or two to take the edge off is normal, but sometimes we spiral out of control. Alcohol cannot bring our loved ones back. It is possible to be a clearheaded griever. My husband was very proud that he died sober, surrounded by those who loved him.

Day Five

"We're all searching for something to fill up what I like to call that big . . . hole in our souls. Some people use alcohol, or sex, or their children, or food, or money, or music, or heroin . . . But it's all the same thing, really. People . . . think they can escape their sorrows."

—TIFFANIE DEBARTOLO

Addictions come in many shapes and sizes. Some, like reading too much, can be fairly harmless. Others can be deadly, harming us physically, financially, emotionally, spiritually. Death leaves a big hole in our soul, in the shape of the one we love who has died. We have to have more, more, more because the hole is bottomless. The only thing that can really begin to fill it is love.

Day Six

"I can't see the logic in medicating a grieving person like there was something wrong with her, and yet it happens all the time . . . We need to walk through our grief, not medicate it and shove it under the carpet like it wasn't there."

—RICHARD WAGNER

Grief can't be medicated away by food, drink, drugs, or even something a doctor prescribes. There may be times in life when medication is useful, but grief is not an illness; it is a normal reaction to death. Grief work entails acknowledging our pain and finding ways to live vibrantly again. Grief work can't be done if we pretend everything is fine.

Day Seven

"I strongly believe that love is the answer and that it can mend even the deepest unseen wounds. Love can heal, love can console, love can strengthen, and yes, love can make change."

—SOMALY MAM

I start every morning with death. Sometimes I read the stories people share on Grief Speaks Out and I cry. What gives me courage is to remember and honor the love. Without love, there is no grief. We can learn to feel the love we were blessed with and to let that love bathe us in light and renewal.

Becoming a Grief Whisperer

Sit down with a stack of paper nearby.

First, think of things you do that are harmful to your mind, body, and spirit. For example, mine would include indulging in fattening foods, lack of exercise, and oversleeping. Now write each thing on separate pieces of paper, using as many pages as you need. If something is a particularly difficult problem you can write it on more than one page. Add one blank page.

Second, think of things you might do to take better care of your mind, body and spirit. Mine might include eating healthy foods, drinking water, exercising, and meditating. Now write each thing on separate pieces of paper, using as many pages as you need. You can include things you might like to try but haven't done yet. Add one blank page.

Now lay both sets of paper down on the floor, each in a completely separate path, Place the blank pages at the end of each path.

Walk the path of harmful behaviors. Be mindful of the sensation of each page as you stand on it. Harmful things often make us feel better, bring us comfort, maybe even have something to teach us. Or they can make us feel awful. When you get to the blank page, stand on it for a while and think of where this path is leading you. How do you feel?

Walk the path of things you might do to take better care of yourself. Be mindful of the sensation of each page as you stand on it. When you get to the blank page at the end, stand on it for a while. Consider where this path is leading you. How do you feel?

The purpose of this exercise is to actively create new patterns in your brain.

Keep the papers and repeat the exercise whenever you wish. You can change the pages in each path as you change. If you ever feel you can give up walking the harmful path you can get rid of those pages. Keep the self-care pages and add to them any time you wish.

Numbness

When your foot falls asleep, you may not want to move for fear of the prickly or sharp pain you will endure until feeling returns. Similarly, it is normal to react to a great loss by going numb, a reaction to the fear of feeling again. Even years later, we can wear our numbness as a cloak to protect us from pain. But by blocking pain, we are also blocking joy.

Day One

> "Now something so sad has hold of us that the breath leaves and we can't even cry."
>
> —CHARLES BUKOWSKI

Sometimes people feel badly because they cry too often. Sometimes people feel badly because they don't cry at all. But tears come when they will. I used to be afraid that if I cried, my tears would never stop. But they did. Then they started again. In time, I found I could remain dry-eyed or cry in ways that better served my emotional needs.

Day Two

"The body shuts down when it has too much to bear; goes its own way quietly inside, waiting for a better time, leaving you numb and half alive."

—JEANETTE WINTERSON

Shutting down when we're under stress is normal. The very definition of grieving is bearing the unbearable. Will a better time to feel deeply again come naturally, or must we look for ways to create it?

Day Three

"I felt very still and empty, the way the eye of a tornado must feel, moving dully along in the middle of the surrounding hullabaloo."

—SYLVIA PLATH

Sometimes numbness masquerades as peace. It seems as though in the middle of a swirl of emotions, we are calm. A clue that we are actually experiencing numbness of feelings and not peace is that we feel empty. We are not filled or fulfilled in the eye of the storm. We are only pretending to be.

Day Four

"There's the kind of grief that leaves you numb, and the kind . . . that rips your world in half. And then there's another kind of grief that doesn't feel like grief at all. It's like a tiny splinter you don't even know you have until it festers so deep it has nowhere left to go but into your soul. I think that's the hardest kind of grief there is . . . you're hurting but you don't know why."

—BETH HOFFMAN

Numbness is a way of being disconnected. Grief doesn't go away with numbness; we just don't feel it. If we don't feel it, it can begin to infect our body, mind, and soul. This is not a tiny splinter that can be pulled out. However, it is a hurting that can be soothed.

Day Five

"It was as though my mind had become one enormous, anesthetized wound. I thought only, *One day I'll weep for this. One of these days I'll start to cry.*"

—JAMES BALDWIN

Anesthesia numbs physical pain, and when it wears off, pain returns. Even if we have successfully made our minds comfortably numb, we are aware on some level of the sadness to come. If we try to keep our numbness intact, we must fight our natural tendency to feel. If we do not weep now, the tears will build up and eventually break through. Sometimes just holding a box of tissues can give us permission to cry.

Day Six

"Nothing could have been as unfamiliar as this grief . . . this vast landscape of sorrow, emptiness and guilt, in which there were no signposts, and no rules on how to behave. If she weren't so numb, she might be amused by the irony of it all; the first thing she ever had to do without Harry was mourn him."

—NICOLA UPSON

Grief is unfamiliar. We are surprised by the different twists and turns it takes. When we are numb feelings can come through. There is a wry amusement to the fact the only person we want to share our grief with is the person who has died.

Day Seven

"I accepted all this counsel politely, with a glassy smile and a glaring sense of unreality. Many adults seemed to interpret this numbness as a positive sign . . . I wasn't howling aloud or punching my fist through windows or doing any of the things I imagined people might do who felt as I did."

—DONNA TARTT

Sometimes people compliment us on our numbness. They look past our glassy eyes and think we are handling our grief in a healthy way. They do not understand that grief needs to be felt and spoken about. Sometimes howling and punching our fists into walls is what is necessary. If grief is unexpressed, it damages us more, not less. How do we alleviate our numbness? Quickly, like ripping a bandage off? Or slowly, in stages? When you are ready, you will know.

Becoming a Grief Whisperer

Find a comfortable place to sit or lie down. If you like, wear or hold something that belonged to your loved one. Place pictures, writings, and/or items belonging to that person nearby. Set an alarm for 15 minutes. Now, put on an imaginary suit of armor or an imaginary suit of soft material that has the power to defend you from emotional and physical harm. Feeling safe and cozy, let your mind go blank. If your thoughts race in a way that disturbs you, repeat anything that allows you to feel safe. It could simply be the word "safe." Repeating something of your choice blocks other thoughts from coming in. Feel free to stop before the alarm goes off.

Now, sit up and look at the pictures and other items you have beside you. Keep your imaginary protective covering on, or experiment with taking it off. You may find yourself feeling sadness or anger or joy or other emotions when looking at and touching these things—let the emotions flow through you, or ask them to go away. You can even return to your meditative, safe position. Experiment, when you are ready, with removing your imaginary protective covering. You can always put it back on. Numbness protects us. You can learn when it is useful and when it is not.

Exhaustion

Grief is exhausting. The trauma of having someone we love die doesn't happen at a fixed time in the past. It happens every morning when we wake up and remember. It happens during the day when things happen that we want to share and cannot. It happens at night when we are about to go to sleep without our loved ones. We can and will develop tools to help us deal with this recurring trauma. We must spend a certain amount of energy living with the fact every day that our loved ones can't come back. How do we generate enough energy to cope with that fact and also to live our lives with passion and joy?

Day One

"People say what doesn't kill you makes you stronger . . . But it doesn't. It breaks your bones, leaving everything splintered . . . Fragile and exhausting to hold together. Sometimes you wish it had killed you."

—FIONA BARTON

Trying to hold our splintered, shattered selves together is exhausting. Even after so many years, I still need time for it all to collapse and fall apart before I can reassemble my parts and start again. Doing this repeatedly doesn't necessarily make us stronger. It may emphasize instead our fragility.

Day Two

"I force myself to think of anything but the one thing that I'm actually always thinking about. And that is so exhausting that I sleep more than I ever have."

—HOLLY GOLDBERG SLOAN

Grief is a thief of energy and time. If I try not to think of my grief, it still forces itself into my consciousness. I may sleep too much to avoid it, and then it enters my dreams.

Day Three

"[She] waited for the night to bring her the same comfort. It didn't . . . she was now too exhausted to sleep—and too heartbroken to weep."

—DIANE SETTERFIELD

Sometimes grief results in the inability to sleep. Sleep deprivation causes even more exhaustion. It seems illogical, but the nature of grief is in itself illogical. We need sleep and are too tired to have the comfort of it. We need to cry, and some of us cry too much but others of us can't cry at all.

Day Four

"I was perishing from exhaustion. I was worn and miserable and I loved crying . . . I gave in to it fully. I felt that profound release of the utterly grief-stricken. I didn't give a damn who saw or heard. I cried and cried."

—ANNE RICE

When I am exhausted from living each moment without my husband, sometimes my tears come from deep within my heart and soul. It's cathartic. In the beginning, tears would spill from my tired eyes wherever I was. Now, I usually cry at home alone, but still, even at unexpected moments, the tears come.

Day Five

"She was tranquil, but it was with the quietness of exhausted grief, not of resignation; and she looked back upon the past, and awaited the future, with a kind of out-breathed despair."

—ANN RADCLIFFE

It's odd that some people think exhausted grief-stricken despair is tranquility. We are too tired to move or speak, and our silent stillness is interpreted as a kind of peace. We may even interpret it this way ourselves. It is too exhausting to feel, so we just stop.

Day Six

"I managed to look like a normal person. I walked the street; I answered my phone; I brushed my teeth, most of the time. But I was not OK. I was in grief. Nothing seemed important. Daily tasks were exhausting . . . At one point I did not wash my hair for ten days."

—MEGHAN O'ROURKE

When my husband first died, daily tasks were so exhausting that I set myself a chore of the day. I would do just one thing so I could go to sleep at night with a feeling of accomplishment. It might be paying one bill or washing one dish. I thought, when I am less tired I can do more.

Day Seven

"I'm tired of being enclosed here. I'm wearying to escape into that glorious world, and to be always there: not seeing it dimly through tears . . . but really with it, and in it."

—EMILY BRONTË

Even in the deepest exhaustion, our life force pulses just beneath the surface. We can be tired of being alive, but also weary of being dead while we are alive. How do we escape from the prison of our grief and find the energy to be with the world, in the world? We may have already started but are still too exhausted to notice the changes we are making.

Becoming a Grief Whisperer

Grief is exhausting. The more tired you are, the more tired you become. I want you to start moving. It could be as simple as moving your little finger or standing up and stretching. It could be as complicated as training for a marathon or learning how to dance. You can do this by yourself in your home. You can take a class or go to the gym. You can take a walk around the block or on a nature trail. You can swim or go shopping. The only thing you need to do is start. When you are ready, give yourself a daily goal: as little as 10 minutes or as much as two hours. Track your progress each day.

Check with your doctor before radically changing an exercise routine.

Anger

One good thing about anger is that it often has energy that despair and depression lack. My husband and I repeated this promise: "Nobody leaves." I know my husband didn't choose to, but I'm still angry at him for leaving me. I want him here with me in his earthly body. The feeling of anger can be intensified in cases of death by suicide, murder, and random accidents. In the beginning, I was also angry at those who had what I had lost. I hated happy couples. I hated anyone over the age my husband was when he died. In some ways, this anger generalized into anger at the whole world. Without my husband's love to buffer my experience of life, I am a much grumpier person. You can call me "Malcontenta."

Day One

"I am angry about what caused you to die. I want to shake my fist or scream at the caregivers who did not save your life . . . It upsets me that you left this world even though I still needed you."

—LINDA ANDERSON

I understand that cancer killed my husband. The doctor that misdiagnosed him took away his chance to fight. I am angry at myself for not recognizing his cancer sooner. I thought his looks changed because he was aging. I am angry at losing him and I accept my anger. I am working on expressing my anger more carefully. Sometimes I snap at people who don't deserve it, and I am trying to stop doing that.

Day Two

"We usually know more about suppressing anger than feeling it . . . Find ways to get it out without hurting yourself or someone else . . . Do not bottle up anger inside. Instead, explore it. The anger is just another indication of the intensity of your love."

—ELISABETH KÜBLER-ROSS

We don't have to pretend that we aren't angry. We can find a safe place to express it, explore it, and learn from it. I don't know who I would be without my anger. It helps me to know the intensity of my anger is due to the intensity of my love. For me, it is merely a question of whether my anger controls me or whether I have learned to control it.

Day Three

"It is possible to be angry with someone who has died. It is possible to hate yourself for being angry with someone who has died . . ."

—ANITA SHREVE

I have been very angry at my husband for dying. I have shouted at him. Then I think, *it wasn't his fault*. But still, I am angry. Could I have stopped him from dying if I had figured out what was wrong? No. I know now that anger isn't rational. It just is.

Day Four

"I knew it wasn't fair, I knew it was wrong, but I couldn't help it. And after a while, the anger I felt just sort of became part of me, like it was the only way I knew how to handle the grief."

—NICHOLAS SPARKS

There is nothing fair about someone we love dying. Whether they are young or old, sick or well, they are our loved ones and we want them to be alive with us. Anger is a way many handle grief. Anger at life, anger at fate, anger that spreads out and touches everything.

Day Five

"Some put on a brave face for others. Others let it all out at once and shatter . . . Then there are the ones like me, where grief is a badge we wear . . . We are the furious ones, the ones that scream at the injustice and the pain . . . "

—T.J. KLUNE

Someone once called me a "radical griever." They were acknowledging my refusal to let go of my grief, wearing it as a badge of love found and love lost. I am furious that my husband has unwillingly left me behind, but it is living in our love that allows me some measure of peace.

Day Six

"Grief is not necessarily any prettier than death, and the grief-stricken do not wander like lambs grateful for the shepherd's guidance. They can be more like wounded wolves, snapping at those who would help them."

—PIERS ANTHONY

Grief can be like someone tap-dancing on one's last nerve. It is difficult not to snap at those who try to help. I apologize often for meeting kindness with rage, but it still happens more than it should. Part of grief work is the gentling down and redirecting of our anger.

Day Seven

"Perhaps grief is like battle: After experiencing enough of it, your body's instincts take over. When you see it closing in like a Martial death squad, you harden your insides . . . You prepare for the agony of a shredded heart. When it hits, it hurts, but not as badly . . . because all that's left is anger and strength."

—SABAA TAHIR

There is strength in anger. There is even more strength in anger that has been tamed. That is my goal: not to never be angry again, but to use my anger as a weapon against grief. I am a grief warrior, and anger is one of the tools I use to emerge not vanquished, but victorious.

Becoming a Grief Whisperer

I found it difficult to express my anger as myself. I had to give myself permission to speak what I was feeling. I needed to create a character to say what I would not. I called mine THE BEAST. You would not believe the things THE BEAST says. I would never say those things! Take time to imagine, or draw, what your angry alter ego looks like. Then, alone or with a trusted friend or therapist, schedule time to give expression to that part of you. You can yell, hit pillows, draw, curse, write, hit drums—anything that suits, but keep your emotional and physical safety in mind. If you feel anger taking over at other times, thank it for showing up and ask it to step aside until it is time for you to pay attention to it and what it is trying to tell you.

Gratitude

Grief can cloud gratitude; it can make us feel that there are no blessings left. But gratitude still exists in us, little seedlings buried beneath winter's frost. Gratitude needs to be nourished. I find gratitude in the time I spend with my loved ones. I find it in the world. In my darkest moments I can be grateful for indoor plumbing. I might think there is nothing left for me to be grateful for. I stop, listen, look and breathe. I discover I am grateful for elephants who mourn their dead, theater, laughter, warm blankets, and all of you who are walking this path with me.

Day One

"And so I have to say that another of the golden threads is gratitude. I was grateful because I knew, even in my fear and grief, that my life had been filled with gifts."

—WENDELL BERRY

The greatest gift of all is the love my husband and I share. In the depth of my grief, I feel that life gives me many colored threads. It is my job to weave them into a rope to pull myself up from the depths of despair. It hurts sliding down again, but even with rope burn, I keep pulling myself up. Gratitude acknowledges the many gifts we are given if we open our hearts to see them while still honoring our pain and suffering.

Day Two

"Gratitude is medicine for a heart devastated by tragedy. If you can only be thankful for the blue sky, then do so."

—RICHELLE E. GOODRICH

I'm more likely to be grateful for a stormy sky. I like the outside world to resemble how I feel inside. As you practice gratitude, begin by finding just one thing to be grateful for, and let the medicine of your gratitude for that one thing start to work. If we can place our gratitude in the time we spent with our loved ones, or seeing a butterfly, or tasting something sweet, it can push aside the sadness for that moment. Each moment of gratitude is a healing salve for the woundedness of grief.

Day Three

"I am always saddened by the death of a good person. It is from this sadness that a feeling of gratitude emerges . . . a reminder to me that my time on this beautiful earth is limited and that I should seize the opportunity to forgive, share, explore, and love."

—STEVE MARABOLI

I want to show my gratitude to my husband, and to all the people I have known and known about, by making my life as rich as I can. One small step at a time, when I am ready. If I can enjoy something, or help another person, I am honoring my dead.

Day Four

"Grief can destroy you—or focus you. You can decide a relationship was all for nothing if it had to end in death, and you alone. OR you can realize that every moment of it had more meaning than you dared to recognize . . . you're driven to your knees not by the weight of the loss but by gratitude for what preceded the loss."

—DEAN KOONTZ

One of the biggest turning points in my grief was when I realized that it was important to me to make my husband's life matter more than his death. I honor him daily by making myself available to other grieving people as he, a recovering alcoholic, made himself available to other addicts. My husband loved life. I honor him daily by finding ways to love life. His smile and his love continue through me. Gratitude lessens the weight of my grief.

Day Five

"There is nothing that can replace the absence of someone dear to us, and one should not even attempt to do so . . . For to the extent the emptiness truly remains unfilled one remains connected to the other person through it . . . the more beautiful and full the remembrances, the more difficult the separation. But gratitude transforms the torment of memory into silent joy."

—DIETRICH BONHOEFFER

There is a blessing in the emptiness because it is a space that belongs only to our dead. The emptiness is our connection, our love. Gratitude blunts the pain of memory and restores its joy.

Day Six

"You will live in me always. Your words, your heart, your soul are all part of me. My heart is full of your memories. Thank you for the gift of your life. I will never forget you."

—AMY ELDON

We are the keeper of our loved ones' stories. They live in us and through us. If we can be grateful for the gift of their lives, for all they have given us, a new feeling can grow. It is still a grief, but a grief with a smile. Grief can have great sadness but also be a vessel for joy. I will never forget you. I love you. You're my heart. Always.

Day Seven

" . . . Because of you I stop to look up at the moon and wish upon a star . . . Because of you I have a broken heart but I thank God for sending you to me. For there is no stronger love than I hold for you."

—MELISSA ESHLEMAN

What do I have in my life, in my heart, because of my beloved dead? The list is long. I learned so much from you, and I continue to be guided by you. Because of you I have resilience, I have appreciation of beauty, I know I am lovable.

Becoming a Grief Whisperer

Gather photos of your loved one. You may also get cards or letters they have written you and any videos you have of them. Spend some time with these things and think of ways you are grateful for them in your life. Now list all the things you are grateful for in the time you spent with your loved one. Make your own "Because of You" list. How is your life enriched by having the gift of loving this person?

Friends and Family: Supportive, Unkind, or Simply Gone?

It is normal to have family and friends give us support. It is unfortunately also normal to have family and friends treat us unkindly or even disappear. It is difficult to grieve for more lost relationships at a time when we are so vulnerable. After my husband died, my oldest, dearest friend stopped speaking to me. Grief does strange things to the griever, but also to those around them. My daughter was always supportive. One friend took my time of grief to renew our relationship. Many of my friends are people I have met since my husband died. There is room for both endings and beginnings.

Day One

"When we ask ourselves which person in our lives mean the most to us, we often find that it is those who, instead of giving advice, solutions, or cures, have chosen rather to share our pain . . . that is a friend who cares . . ."

—HENRI J.M. NOUWEN

I have found the dearest people are those who don't try to fix me. I don't want to be fixed. Unless you can bring my husband back to life, there is nothing you can really do. I am lucky to have people who listen, who sit with me in grief, with acknowledgment and acceptance. I try to do that for others. I make a space for them to feel free to talk about their beloved dead while I listen.

Day Two

"[She] would much rather have imaginary friends who were real than real friends who were imaginary."

—REBECCA MCNUTT

I value honesty and authenticity above all things. Some people who I thought were real friends were imaginary. I cannot say if they loved me once and changed, or if they were always imaginary. If you are not going to be a real friend, please don't be a friend at all.

Day Three

"Step two of the Great Grief Showcase: I Knew Him Better Than You. Whoever is being carted off to the morgue is now becoming best friends with dozens of people . . . because that intimacy will bump them up higher on the grieving pecking order. Their tears will hurt more, their lives will matter more because a bigger hole has been torn into it by this untimely, tragic death."

—S.G. REDLING

We can never measure our grief against another person's grief. Grief is not a competitive sport. Some people might make their grief bigger, more important than ours. People can be hurtful and awkward when confronted with grief. Know that you are not alone in experiencing this.

Day Four

"The dirty secret she'd learned about grief was that nobody wanted to hear about your loss a week after the funeral. People you'd once considered friends would turn their heads in church or cross to another side of a shopping mall to avoid the contamination of your suffering."

—SUSAN DORMADY EISENBERG

Grief is one of the most overwhelming, powerful, misunderstood emotions. It makes people uncomfortable. Here we are, walking examples of the fact that life isn't perfect. People we love die and our world is shattered. It is so painful, yet so ordinary, to be ignored by those whose comfort we so deeply need.

Day Five

"I wasn't showing what I really felt. Real grief is ugly and uncomfortable. People look away from grief the same way they look away from severed limbs or gaping wounds. What they want is pain like death on a stage: beautiful, bloodless, presented for their entertainment."

—SARAH REES BRENNAN

As unusually open as I am about my grief, I still keep the darkest moments a secret. I don't want to frighten people and I don't want to hear their advice. I know how many people want to look away from grief, which means away from who I really am. It can add to the griever's sense of alienation. How much is safe to share and how much should remain hidden is difficult to measure.

Day Six

"What's even more messed up than funerals, is the way people treat you after the funeral. Like you're diseased or something."

—DENISE JADEN

Many people attended the celebration of my husband's life. People even flew in from great distances to be there for me. Some were there for a short time. Some were never there. The precious ones are still there whenever I need them. After a funeral is when we learn who our friends truly are. People can lose patience with our continuing grief. Grief is not a disease. It is not contagious. I wish people would not try to put grievers into quarantine.

Day Seven

"Community is about sharing my life; about allowing the chaos of another's circumstances to infringe on mine . . . about resigning myself to needing others."

—SANDY OSHIRO ROSEN

My circle of friends today is different than it once was. My friends today know I will talk about my husband when I want to. There are some old friends still, but many are new ones. One of my dearest friends is someone I have known for only a short while. One of the things that binds us together is our grief and our connection to our beloved dead. I am grateful for those who stand with me in my grief and allow this loner to be a part of a community.

Becoming a Grief Whisperer

Buy two candles: a thick or sturdy one that will take a long time to burn, and a smaller one that will burn quickly, like a tea light. Light the larger candle and thank anyone who has stood by you and supported you. If you don't have anyone who has done this, ask the burning light to bring people into your life who will be there for you. Now light the smaller candle and say whatever you need to say to the people who have hurt you or abandoned you. Watch the little candle disappear while the big candle continues to give light and warmth.

Guilt

Some grievers feel guilty, because we are still alive and the person we love has died. We feel guilty because we couldn't protect our loved one and keep them from dying. We feel guilty because we are having a good day and smiling and laughing, and that seems disloyal. We feel guilty because we feel guilty. When I look into my husband's remembered eyes, I see love and forgiveness. Can I feel that love and forgiveness for myself in my own heart?

Day One

> "Even when you are happy to see your friends again and laugh at their jokes, the relief is mixed with sadness and, maybe, guilt."
>
> —ELISABETH KÜBLER-ROSS

It's normal to feel guilty whenever grief subsides. We link honor and remembrance with sadness and pain. It took me a few years to realize I wanted to make my husband's life more important than his death, and that it was my responsibility to live double now; for him and for me.

Day Two

"The spaces between the times you miss them grow longer. Then, when you do remember to miss them again, it's still with a stabbing pain to the heart. And you have guilt. Guilt because it's been too long since you missed them last."

—KRISTIN O'DONNELL TUBB

Are there moments when we don't miss our loved ones? For me, the missing is always there, but sometimes it is conscious and sometimes it goes underground. It is normal to reengage with life and have the longing become less acute. If you realize that the missing's not gone, perhaps that can lessen guilt.

Day Three

"Grief is an ocean, and guilt the undertow that pulls me beneath the waves and drowns me."

—SHAUN DAVID HUTCHINSON

We can drown in grief and in guilt. Guilt can take over our lives. As we tame our grief, perhaps we can learn to also tame our guilt.

Day Four

"I felt bad for trying to live a happy, full life, while my heart was buried in a dead man's chest."

—KRISTEN HOPE MAZZOLA

I think my heart is still buried in a dead man's chest. My heart is also still beating. I have a letter from my husband telling me how proud he is of me because when I fall down, I get back up again and keep trying. I still want him to be proud of me. Perhaps a happy life is a sign of proper grieving just as much as a sad life is.

Day Five

"You feel sick with guilt . . . You can't remember anything thoughtful or sweet or tender thing that you ever did even though logically you know you must have. All you can recall is how often you were small and petty and false . . . "

—ELAN MASTAI

It's normal to feel guilty about all the things you could have said and done. There is so much wasted time in so many relationships. I want a do-over. I want us to have a chance, not to love each other more, but to show it more. When I get stuck in this way of thinking, I am learning to remember all the special moments we did share, all the sweet and loving things we said and did. If we had been perfect, we would not have been human.

Day Six

"Guilt is sneaky. It is powerful and relentless. It accomplishes nothing. It is not our friend . . . but guilt is so familiar. We get its voice confused with our own. Beating ourselves up becomes as natural as breathing."

—GARY ROE

There are so many things I wish I had done better. I'm not sure I can forgive myself, but my husband already has. I will let him guide me, even now.

Day Seven

"The problem with surviving was that you ended up with the ghosts of everyone you'd ever left behind riding on your shoulders."

—PAOLO BACIGALUPI

Here's the thing: I like my ghosts. I love my ghosts. I can be guilty that I am alive and they are dead and find their weight on my shoulders crippling, or I can be grateful to have a life full of love even if loss came with it. My surviving will not last forever. Someday I will join my ghosts and we will ride together.

Becoming a Grief Whisperer

Take out a picture of yourself as a baby or at any young age. If you don't have any pictures, imagine yourself at that age. How would you care for that little baby? What would be your hopes and dreams for that little baby? That small innocent being is you, the you that still needs loving care. Say to the picture, "I forgive you." Take a deep breath in and exhale. Say, "I forgive myself." If you want, touch the picture gently. You don't have to believe it. Try saying "I forgive myself," as an experiment and see how you feel.

Now take a picture of your loved one and look into their eyes. Imagine them saying, "I forgive you. I want you to live in happiness and peace," or substitute your own words. When guilt comes, look at yourself through your loved one's remembered eyes. Hear them again saying, "I forgive you. I want you to live in happiness and peace." You can even imagine your loved one saying, "We will be together soon, and I want you to have so many stories to share with me."

Intimacy

When someone you love dies, you lose the comfort of both emotional and physical intimacy. I had an emotional closeness with my husband that I have never had with anyone else. We had shared history and private jokes that no one else would get. Some people think of physical intimacy as something erotic or sexual in nature, but physical intimacy is also touch; for example, the way a child and a parent hold each other. When my husband died, I lost my back scratcher and my foot rubber. I once said to him, "Thank you for holding me." A rather tough guy, he replied, "I need it as much as you do."

Day One

"Her absence is like the sky, spread over everything . . . There is one place where her absence comes locally home to me, and it is a place I can't avoid. I mean my own body."

—C.S. LEWIS

When my husband and I curled into each other, I called the way we fit "my nooks and crannies." My husband's absence is everywhere. No one else was attuned to his body the way I was. My mind can be filled in many ways, but my body feels empty.

Day Two

> "Terrifying, that the loss of intimacy with one person results in the freezing over of the world, and the loss of oneself."

—JAMES BALDWIN

When your being is interconnected with another being it is difficult not to feel the loss of oneself with the loss of them. Being interdependent is not the same as being codependent. I always said my husband held my kite string so I could soar. Now even though there are many other people in the world it is a much colder place.

Day Three

> "You lose her in pieces over a long time—the way the mail stops coming, and her scent fades from the pillows . . . Just when the day comes . . . that overwhelms you with the feeling that she's gone, forever—there comes another day, and another specifically missing part."

—JOHN IRVING

The truth is that even when someone is old or ill we never expect their death. Not that day. We keep noticing things we miss. So much is gone forever and cannot be replaced that we cannot absorb it all at once. Each new day can bring "another specifically missing part."

Day Four

"She doesn't want another body, she wants the body she loved."

—MICHELLE LATIOLAIS

Earthly love is physical as well as emotional and spiritual. I love walking with my granddaughter's hand in mine. Another child's hand will not do; it must be my granddaughter's hand. People often expect us to find solace elsewhere. We can find other loves. Many people do. That does not mean we stop aching for our loved ones.

Day Five

"She remembered . . . reaching across the bed every morning when she woke up for eight years expecting to find him there . . . and only slowly growing accustomed to the fact that that side of the bed would always be empty. The moments when she had found something funny and turned to share the joke with him, only to be shocked anew that he was not there."

—CASSANDRA CLARE

What is the part of me that is still surprised that you are not here? Sometimes I feel silly. It's been over eight years, and every day I wonder how it is possible that you are not going to come home. People talk about acceptance. For most grievers, there is always a part of them that never fully accepts a death. Even if our mind accepts it, our body does not.

Day Six

"But those two circles, above all the point at which they touched, are the very thing I am mourning for . . . You tell me 'she goes on.' But my heart and body are crying out, come back, come back. Be a circle, touching my circle on the plane of Nature . . . "

—C.S. LEWIS

That is the silent cry of all grievers. Whether you believe in an afterlife or not, it is natural to want the person you love to be here now. We are two circles, always touching, but now one circle is in a place I cannot see or touch with my physical being. I live each day knowing that what I most want, what I most need is impossible.

Day Seven

"Since he died some of the [colors] have disappeared. I have lost the violet of seeing him, the indigo of touching him . . . But I can still see . . . the red of the feelings in my heart, the orange of his possessions, the yellow of our memories . . . Sometimes I lose sight even of these [colors]. I search in the shadows, hungry for another glimpse, desperate that I may have lost them forever. This is my darkness."

—THOMAS HARDING

Many people describe grief as having "drained the color" out of their life. The black darkness is the absence of color. The question is always, "How do I retain a sense of intimacy with someone who is no longer breathing, who no longer has a body?" It's not easy loving a dead person. Yet, I believe love is eternal.

Becoming a Grief Whisperer

To relieve the stress of the loss of physical intimacy, consider things you can do to take care of your body. Have you tried massage, Reiki, chiropractic, or other body work? At home, you can try body creams or bubble baths. Does it help to hold a pillow when you sleep?

To relieve the loss of emotional intimacy, we are lucky if we have people we can share things with. However, our loved ones can still be communicated with. Every night or morning, write a letter to your loved one. Write about your hopes and dreams and anything else you want to share. Ask their advice and listen for a response.

As far as experiencing intimacy with a new person, there is no wrong or right answer to when or if this is appropriate. Some grievers take solace in other relationships; others do not. It is something to ponder with gentleness and patience.

Abandonment

There are different kinds of abandonment. Sometimes people we thought we could count on abandon us. Sometimes we feel that the person who died abandoned us. Sometimes we feel abandoned by our beloved dead when, except in the tragic case of suicide, we know that death wasn't something they chose. Sometimes we feel abandoned by God or our higher power. Our prayers were not answered the way we wanted. The sense of abandonment is common. It can intensify other feelings.

Day One

"There are far too many silent sufferers. Not because they don't yearn to reach out, but because they've tried and found no one who cares."

—RICHELLE E. GOODRICH

I have always refused to be silent, but I understand why others make that choice. People need a safe space where they can speak openly and have their feelings supported. Grieving is difficult enough without having to also grieve for lost friendships and people's lack of concern.

Day Two

"'How could you leave me?' she cried out loud . . . She wanted to kick the gravestone; she wanted to tear out the earth beneath which her mother lay and pull the body out of the ground and shake it until it gave her an answer."

—MALINDA LO

"How could you leave me?" is now a question with no answer. Even if we could dig our loved ones up, we would not have them with us. My husband is not in his ashes, yet his ashes are all I have left of his physical self. How can I begin to accept that, even without wanting to, he has left me?

Day Three

"I'd suffered many losses in recent years . . . In her final years my mother often lamented that there was no one alive who had known her as a girl and I was starting to understand how spooked she'd felt. I wasn't sure I could take any more abandonments."

—DIANE ACKERMAN

I was at a funeral, and a man I didn't know wandered up to me and said, "There is no one left." It is difficult to have one person die, but so many people have lost more than one. We feel we can't take any more abandonments, and then we do.

Day Four

> "You are really alone, especially if you are abandoned by those who were supposed to care for you."
>
> —BANGAMBIKI HABYARIMANA

I am lucky to have many friends. However, having so many people I thought would always care for me stop speaking to me makes me feel alone. I am less close to people than I once was. This is part of my grief work. In order to have the benefits of closeness I will have to become willing to risk loss.

Day Five

> "The one who dies has it easy, you know. The one who's left behind is the one who truly suffers."
>
> —D.T. DYLLIN

There is a phrase that some people find helpful and others find infuriating, "They are in a better place." To them I say, wherever the better place is, they are still not here. It is we who must learn to live without them. It is a gift we give to those we love who have gone before; that we grieve for them so they do not have to grieve for us.

Day Six

"I woke up to an ache in my chest . . . the smell of chocolate, and the sound of the ghost making a racket in the kitchen. I think my heart is smart enough to know there's a place I should be filling with new memories . . . But that person is gone now. And so, my heart has a giant hole. I call it The Big Empty."

—NATALIE LLOYD

My life is full and empty. I have made many new memories. Nothing hurts more than knowing I cannot make new memories with the one person I want to make them with most of all. I love my ghost. I wish he would make more of a racket.

Day Seven

"Those we love never truly leave us. There are things that death cannot touch."

—JACK THORNE

In the midst of abandonment, pain, and loss, I truly believe that love triumphs over death. When I think of death I am sad, but then I think of love and I am grateful. Perhaps I only feel abandoned. Perhaps my husband never left. Not in the way that matters: love.

Becoming a Grief Whisperer

Close your eyes and imagine (or draw a picture, or write a story) your loved one has come back to you. What does it feel like to have them with you? Are you walking on a beach or sitting quietly and telling stories? Are you yelling at them for leaving you? Ask them how they might suggest you can feel them with you. If you imagine what your loved one would say, or even make something up, this can be another way of communicating. If you believe that it is not right to speak to someone who has died, then you can just use your imagination. You knew and loved this person—you can guess what they would say. If your loved one took their own life, be extra gentle with yourself while doing this exercise.

Faith

Grief can strengthen faith. Grief can destroy faith. As we change, our faith can change. We can have faith in a particular God, but also in goddesses, nature, the life force, or even oneself. Faith defies logic. In asking where we can go for comfort, many people find faith is the answer. If you feel your faith has been shaken or lost, remember what has been lost can be found. One who has wandered away can return.

Day One

"Some nights in the midst of this loneliness I swung among the scattered stars at the end of the thin thread of faith alone."

—WENDELL BERRY

There is nothing lonelier than the death of someone central to our very existence. But there are always threads to hold on to, to pull us back to life. When all other threads have shredded, sometimes the strongest one is our faith.

Day Two

"In the Old Testament, a person in grief tore his robe . . . There was weeping and wailing. But in our nutty society, the person who 'keeps it together,' who's 'so brave,' and who 'looks so great—you'd never know,' that's who is applauded. Grief is not the opposite of faith. Mourning is not the opposite of hope."

—JENNIFER SAAKE

I have heard from some grievers that they were told by men and women of faith that if they are grieving they are not true believers and that true believers must always be joyous. This is hurtful and is not based on accurate interpretation of religious principles. If we find someone of our faith who is not patient and loving with our grief, we must look for someone who is.

Day Three

"In the midst of the darkness of loss, I found light . . . As I stumbled over the roots of hopelessness and despair, that light grew to illuminate my path, a path I sometimes felt very alone on. At some point in the journey I'd turned around, and there was God. That is grace."

—MARY POTTER KENYON

There is always light. Grief may blind us to it, but it remains. If you sense even a small spark of light, pay attention to it. Nurture it and wait for it to grow stronger. Faith lights the darkness. Grace shows us the way home.

Day Four

"Grief is a winding, nasty road that has no predictable course, and the best thing you can do as a friend is to show up for the ride. You cannot rush grief . . . "

—ANGIE SMITH

Grief starts as an imbalance. The pain is great and hope seems impossible. As time passes, it may or may not heal, but you may feel the balance shifting. The time it takes to find the joy in the anguish is not known. Months are normal; years are normal. You may find a kind of balance between hope and pain, and then it all shifts again.

Day Five

"Be near as we are surrounded by this cloud of deep suffering . . . Wrap us up inside of the cloud and reveal the mysteries that can only be learned in places of sorrow . . . that . . . we will be . . . transformed by the shadow and beaming radiant light. Give us the strength to love on, though our hearts are broken."

—ANNA WHITE

Part of grief work is to be transformed by shadow into a vessel that holds even more radiant light. Can we continue to love even though our hearts are broken? Can we, as living human beings, afford not to love? May the answer to this prayer be blessings you once thought impossible.

Day Six

"You cussed. Sooner or later, every curse is a prayer."

—TERRY PRATCHETT

I once heard Elie Wiesel say that if you curse God, it is a prayer, because you are still talking. Sometimes we think we have lost our faith but it is our anger hiding it. When the sun is behind a dark cloud, it still shines brightly. Sometimes we lose our faith, and we have to decide if we are content with the loss or if there is a spiritual practice that might help us regain it.

Day Seven

"My faith never wavers that each dear friend I have 'lost' is a new link between this world and the happier land beyond the morn . . . the light of faith never fades from the sky, and I take heart again, glad they are free. "

—HELEN KELLER

How beautiful to have faith in a connection that lives on. Death ends life as we know it but love continues. I, too, take that chance. I believe that our loved ones are still with us. I believe that continuing to remember them with joy and tenderness is a gift I will not refuse. My relationship with my dead is not denial; it is what gives me the strength to be fully alive with grief.

Becoming a Grief Whisperer

Write your own prayer. It can be religious or secular, depending on your beliefs. You can write a prayer of praise, a request for blessings, or a prayer of want and need. It can also be a prayer of questions or anger. When you are satisfied with your message, pick a time each day to read your prayer out loud or to yourself. You can write as many prayers as you wish. You can also decorate them with many colors or even gold or silver leaf. Please read a prayer you have written once each day. It can be the same prayer, or it can change as you change.

No One Understands How I Feel

Grief's loneliness can be deepened by the feeling that no one understands how we feel. So many grievers remain silent due to their sense of privacy or fear of being hurt, that it's difficult to find others who can help us step out of our isolation and help us realize that we are not crazy; we are doing and feeling things many grievers do and feel. There is a rather unkind thing I do to people who are persistent in misunderstanding my grief. I say simply, "Pretend you just answered your phone. You received the terrible message that your loved one is dead. When will you get over it?" In response, I have seen tough men cry.

Day One

"Though I knew in my mind that others had felt such loss, this loss was mine, and I felt that no one would ever understand it, and to try to explain the loneliness and pain I felt would be futile."

—LINDA HAWLEY

Just as each person is unique, each person's experience of grief is unique. Although it is meant to comfort, one of the worst platitudes is, "I know how you feel." No, you don't. Only I know how I feel. Many people may grieve for the person who is our dearest beloved. We still have a special relationship with them. Only we understand how special that relationship is.

Day Two

"People think they know you . . . They don't know what's going on inside your head—the mind-numbing cocktail of anger and sadness and guilt . . . And so they pretend and they say you're doing great when you're really not. And this makes everyone feel better. Everybody but you."

—WILLIAM H. WOODWELL JR.

I hide the times when I shout into the night, "I hate my life. I can't stand this." I hide the times when the tears still come, raw and raging. People don't realize that after so many years, grief still takes its toll. Feeling that my grief has ended makes others feel better; it makes me feel worse.

Day Three

"Every broken heart has screamed at one time or another: Why can't you see who I truly am?"

—SHANNON L. ALDER

It's normal to want to remain hidden. It is also normal to want to be seen. The fear is that if we are seen, we will not be loved. Sometimes this has already come true—we're open to someone we trust and they turn away. I want you to see who I truly am, in my wholeness and brokenness, and I want you to love me even when you see the tattered me.

Day Four

> "Usually when you are grieving someone says something so senselessly optimistic to you, it's about them. Either they want to feel like they can say something helpful, or they simply cannot allow themselves to entertain the finality and pain of death, so they turn it into a Precious Moments greeting card."
>
> —NADIA BOLZ-WEBER

One way to forgive people saying carelessly unkind things is to think that they mean well—they are trying to bring comfort. This can also be hurtful and irritating. Optimism can be as ignorant of grief as pessimism. People who have the courage to look at grief and grievers with open eyes and an honest heart are those who give us authentic precious moments.

Day Five

> "What do you know of the griefs that are in me and what do I know of yours? And if I were to cast myself down before you and weep and tell you, what more would you know about me?"
>
> —FRANZ KAFKA

As no one understands me, so I do not understand them. The person before me with the smiling face and laughing eyes might be concealing the deepest grief. I cannot truly explain my grief; I can only suggest its true nature. As difficult as it may be, I ask for patience for others. I ask for understanding and the capacity for compassion and love, because I do not know the measure of their suffering.

Day Six

"Grief isolates, and every ritual, every gesture, every embrace, is a hopeless effort to break through that isolation. None of it works."

—STEVEN ERIKSON

Words and gestures fail us. Even kindness and a gentle touch fail us. No one can understand how we feel or who we are now. Do we embrace our isolation by retreating into ourselves, or do we accept the part of us that remains unknown and seek community, support, friendship, and even joy in whatever form it now takes?

Day Seven

"Grief is a walk alone. Others can be there, and listen. But you will walk alone down your own path, at your own pace, with your sheared-off pain, your raw wounds, your denial, anger, and bitter loss. You'll come to your own peace, hopefully, but it will be on your own."

—CATHY LAMB

Peace. Loneliness, misunderstanding, pain, anger, bitter loss. Peace. That is the miracle of being fully alive with grief. Peace can be found. Life can be found. In your own way, in your own time. You don't have to let go to move forward. When you are ready.

Becoming a Grief Whisperer

Find a comfortable place to sit or lie down. Play music if you wish. Close your eyes. Create a person or entity that could understand you completely. It could be a higher power or God. It could be a grandparent. It could be a small child. It could be an animal. It could be the person you love who died. It could be a white light. It can be anything that feels right to you. When you have found this fount of understanding, use all your senses to make it come alive. Either silently or with words, let this understanding of you be communicated fully and deeply. Let this understanding be met with unconditional love. When you have spent as much time as you wish being lovingly understood, slowly come back to "real life," and bring the feeling of being understood and loved with you. If you wish, draw a picture of this entity or model it out of clay. Another choice is to carry a small smooth stone or any talisman to remind you of these feelings wherever you are.

The Unbearable Weight of Grief

Grief is not an object, yet it has an ever-shifting shape and weight. Grief feels heavy. Grief feels sharp. It as though our shoulders are stooped now because we carry our grief. We can learn how to change its size and shape so it becomes not just bearable, but useful. What lightens grief? Love.

Day One

"Grief is an unfillable hole in your body. It should be weightless, but it's heavy. Should be cold, but it burns. Should, over time, close up, but instead it deepens."

—EMILY HENRY

In the beginning, my grief was all there was. Its weight was in tons. Over time, the wounds of grief often deepen, but the medicine we learn to apply, when we are ready, can be soothing.

Day Two

"He had forgotten that grief does not decline in a straight line . . . Instead, it was almost as if his body contained a big pile of garden rubbish full both of heavy lumps of dirt and of sharp thorny brush that would stab him when he least expected it."

—HELEN SIMONSON

We can be walking along smiling at the beauty around us and suddenly we double over in pain. Our bodies contain both the heaviness and sharpness of grief. At times we manage to live around it, and then it jolts when we least expect it.

Day Three

"Every morning, I wake up and forget just for a second that it happened. But once my eyes open, it buries me like a landslide of sharp, sad rocks . . . I'm heavy, like there's too much gravity on my heart."

—SARAH OCKLER

I call this sensation "morning mourning." There is that moment when we first open our eyes and are given the blessing of forgetfulness. Then we realize that we have to live once again buried under the landslide of grief. The absence of our loved one is the gravity on our heart.

Day Four

"Grief isn't something you get over. You live with it. You go on with it lodged in you . . . Grief makes me heavy. It makes me slow. Even on days when I laugh a lot, or dance, or finish a project . . . it is there. Lodged deep inside of me."

—ANN HOOD

This is what people who have never experienced great grief fail to understand. We don't "get over" grief. We make it our companion, our partner. Even when we are laughing, dancing, and creating, it is there. Grief can give a certain heaviness to even our lightest moments.

Day Five

"In lieu of letting go of our trauma . . . in my experience, we learn how to carry it and there are some days when it is heavier than others. Some days, I hardly know it is there . . . while other days, the burden is cripplingly heavy and I can hardly breathe under the weight of grief."

—L.M. BROWNING

It is normal to experience shifts in the quality of our grief. There are days we carry it with style and grace. We think we are finally free. Then, sometimes near a birthday or anniversary, or even on an ordinary day, our mouse-sized grief transforms suddenly to a herd of elephants sitting on our chest. We can send them away or lie still and wait for the weight to subside.

Day Six

"We cry in our own rooms, remembering a man who will never be here again. The house creaks. Maybe it feels the weight of our grief, maybe the floorboards are buckling because the burden is too heavy."

—ROCHELLE MAYA CALLEN

Sometimes the weight of grief is also felt in our surroundings. My whole living space is filled with the burden of emptiness. How loud the silence of someone being gone forever echoes. It seems even our most solid surroundings are about to collapse.

Day Seven

"The grief doesn't go away . . . It's like carrying a heavy stone . . . you learn to settle the weight properly, and then you get used to it, and then sometimes you can forget you're carrying it."

—RACHEL NEUMEIER

In time, grief work teaches us how to carry our grief like a model carelessly balances a heavy book on her head. The weight of it becomes more of a caress than a punishment. We are carrying the memory of our loved one and we are carrying love. Our grief muscles have been working out, and they are in less pain than before.

Becoming a Grief Whisperer

This exercise explores the weight of grief. Gather a pile of small rocks that are large enough to write on—from your garden, the seaside, or any other place. You can even purchase them from a garden or craft store.

With a marker or paint, write something about grief that weighs you down on each rock. Some of my words would be sadness, loneliness, and emptiness. Leave some rocks blank. You can also decorate the rocks.

When you have as many rocks as you need, place them in a bag. See how heavy the bag is. Each day, remove one rock or as many as you can. If all the labeled rocks burden you, remove a blank rock. As you feel the bag lighten, you may feel yourself lighten. Keep the rocks somewhere special, and on days when grief feels heavy, place them back in the bag. You can empty the entire bag and imagine what it would feel like if you had no grief left at all.

Wearing a Mask

Many grievers are more comfortable hiding their real selves. They feel vulnerable and pretend they are healing when they are not. They say they're fine when they are far from fine. They do not want to burden others, or hear platitudes, or face once again how little grief is understood or valued. A mask may be hard to wear and sometimes it may slip, but in time, some grievers have a mask for every situation. What they have trouble finding is their own face.

Day One

"People get tired of you bringing it up. People get burdened by your sadness. So you act like it doesn't hurt anymore . . . just so you won't annoy anyone with your grief."

—BRITTAINY C. CHERRY

People can be impatient with grief. I thought I had discovered a good answer to, "How are you?" I would say, "I'm okay with not being okay." Only three weeks after my husband's death, a kind friend asked, "Still?" It becomes easier to pretend that it doesn't hurt anymore—not for yourself, but so you don't bother others.

Day Two

"Like Batman, all of us hide behind our masks and use them to help define ourselves for others. They're not lies, really. They're just not the whole truth, because . . . most of the people we encounter day-to-day couldn't handle the truth (or perhaps we couldn't handle giving it to them)."

—PAUL ASAY

It takes a certain courage and stubbornness to confront people with our raw and honest truth. Can they handle it? Can we handle giving it to them? We think not, so we wear a mask. We give them a false, but in our minds more acceptable, face.

Day Three

"I hide behind a mask . . . I try to reinvent myself. It doesn't work. There are times when I am bone-crushingly sad. I just want to curl into a ball and hide . . . But, I plaster on a smile and play the game for my family and friends."

—JULIA CRANE

In some ways grief continues to imprison us. We could stay home and curl up in a ball and cry. Some of us do. Most of us learn to smile and invent a character for ourselves. The fact that people don't see behind our masks, don't want to see behind our masks, strengthens our sense of isolation. How can they help us escape when they don't even know escape is needed?

Day Four

"Those who suffer intolerably learn to hide their afflictions . . . because the world does not run on pain time but on happy time, whether or not that happiness is honestly felt or a mask for the blackest despondency."

—THOMAS LIGOTTI

"Follow your bliss," they say, choosing false happiness over authenticity. "If you aren't happy," they say, "you are doing it wrong. You are a negative person." Who are they? False prophets. Real mental health is honest expression of feelings. Real friendship is the intimacy that allows for the sharing of truth.

Day Five

"A mask is what we wear to hide from ourselves."

—KHANG KIJARRO NGUYEN

We think our mask is to hide from others, but it is also to hide from ourselves. Do I even know who I am anymore? If I didn't wear a mask to hide from myself, would I disappear under the weight of my emotional, physical, and spiritual pain?

Day Six

"We tend to make adjustments in our lives to get by, to survive. Sometimes we don't actually heal. We make changes. We deny. We mask. We cover up. We hide things . . ."

—SCOTT HILDRETH

Some grievers choose to live with a mask to hide their deepest grief from both themselves and others. We cannot change what hurts us so we don't think of it. We think we are healing when we are only building walls around who we truly are and what we truly feel.

Day Seven

"I look in the mirror and see a person. This person puts on another person's face when she goes out . . . She prefers to be who she is, tries her own person out gradually. She fails most of the time. But the more she does it the better she feels. No more hiding behind the mask. Accept me as I am."

—TINA J. RICHARDSON

Here I am. I am fine, but my husband is still dead, so part of me is not fine. Sometimes I am hidden, but sometimes I am revealed. If you don't like me, that is your choice. Without the mask, I will know who loves and accepts me as I am. If you accept me as I am, I will, in turn, accept you as you are. That is genuine and meaningful love.

Becoming a Grief Whisperer

Play a little game of hide-and-seek with yourself. Buy a mask or make one. You may choose to have several masks with different expressions. If you are comfortable, look into a mirror when you do this exercise. Put the mask over your face. Say something that you say when you are in public. Take the mask off. Now speak the truth. Put the mask back on. Say another thing you say when you are in public. Take the mask off. Again, now speak your real truth. Repeat as many times as you wish. End by saying, No, I am *not* fine, thank you very much. No, I am *not* stuck, thank you very much. No, I don't need you to fix me, thank you very much. No, I am *not* crazy, thank you very much. I am grieving. Everything I do and feel is what normal grieving people do. Feel free to substitute words that work for you.

Mood Swings/Grief Attacks

Mood swings are normal for grievers and can make us hard to live with. There are so many triggers in our environment that send us spiraling in different directions. That is why there are so many names for them. In time we learn to recognize the triggers and hopefully we become less explosive. In my case, when my husband first died, I hated seeing other couples, especially happy ones—especially ones where the man was older than my husband. Now, I love people being in love. Be patient, tender and understanding with yourself even if you can't, right now, find that patience in others.

Day One

"We are not accustomed to the emotional upheaval that accompanies a loss . . . We can go from feeling okay to feeling devastated in a minute without warning. We can have mood swings that are hard for anyone around us to comprehend, because even we don't understand them."

—ELISABETH KÜBLER-ROSS

"Acceptance" may not be acceptance of death, but rather acceptance of your own continuing swirl of emotions in reaction to the death of a loved one. Many grievers feel, or are told, that they are "doing it wrong." One step forward, 300 steps back. It's important to understand that changes in mood—slow or gradual, sudden, up, down, and sideways—are normal.

Day Two

"Grief. I don't know how to describe it other than as a roller coaster that drops you into the pit of hell with the rats and the demons, and then lifts you up above the clouds to the place where heaven begins."

—JESSICA THOMPSON

Grief is an unpredictable roller coaster. There are moments when you feel the pain will never end, and then you are lifted up by love to the place where heaven begins and you feel that you can almost touch your loved one again.

Day Three

"Grieving is like being set afire. Except when you try to put out the flames they disappear; when you try to salve your wounds you find your skin unblemished. You take a breath, thinking the worst has passed, and then grief bursts into flame anew . . . you have no choice but to burn."

—MARSHALL THORNTON

Did you ever throw water on an oily cooking fire only to watch the flames get bigger? That's grief. You don't know when what you have learned will work. The only hope is that the fire will cleanse as well as destroy, leaving room for new growth.

Day Four

"Assassin grief (is) the kind of grief that lies in wait and attacks you from ambush . . . Assassin grief can hide for years and then strike suddenly on the happiest day, without discernible reason or exegesis . . . The enemy is your own grieving heart and, when it strikes, it can't miss."

—GREGORY DAVID ROBERTS

That's what it can feel like. Grief is a sniper or an assassin. It shoots at you when you least expect it, and it seems like there is no armor you can wear, no maneuvers you can make to protect yourself.

Day Five

"Grief slipped away, only to attack from behind. It changed shape endlessly. It lacerated her, numbed her, stalked her, startled her, caught her by the throat . . . Each time [she] escaped her sorrow, forgetful amid other things, she lost him anew the instant she remembered he was gone."

—KATE MALOY

What shape will my grief be today? Will I keep seeing the one I love who died? Will I continue to be surprised that they have died? Will these constant reminders cause so many different feelings that I will never know what is coming next?

Day Six

"People think it's just forgetting your keys, she says. Or the words for things. But there are the personality changes. The mood swings. The hostility and even violence. Even from the gentlest person in the world. You lose the person you love. And you are left with the shell."

—ALICE LAPLANTE

Do you find yourself having more hostility than you had before? Do you find your personality has changed beyond recognition? This is normal. Rebuilding can happen. First there is the empty shell, then there are the pieces we learn to fill the emptiness with. When we are ready.

Day Seven

"And once the storm is over you won't remember how you made it through, how you managed to survive. You won't even be sure, whether the storm is really over. But one thing is certain. When you come out of the storm you won't be the same person who walked in."

HARUKI MURAKAMI

When we come through our storm of grief we are changed. We can find ourselves different in both lovely and horrible ways. Perhaps when the storms come again, as they will, we will have learned how to weather them. There is the possibility of survival. Survival with grace.

Becoming a Grief Whisperer

We often feel the many causes of mood swings and grief attacks are invisible and unexpected and therefore incapable of being prepared for. Place between 5 and 20 sticky notes on a piece of paper. Think of things that might cause a grief attack or mood swing. Write on each sticky note a different possible cause. It might be a song, a date, or time of year. It might be seeing an intact family. It might be something your loved one liked to do. It might be a certain type of food or scent. These will be personal to you. You can always add more sticky notes or take ones away that no long apply.

Underneath each sticky note write anything you can think of that might change how you react to this cause (sometimes called a trigger). You might write "Avoid" or "Accept" under some. Some will need more complex actions. Leave the space blank if you can't think of something right now.

I used to get angry and sad when I saw boxing or tennis, which my husband loved. I decided I would replace saying in my head, "How can they still do that when he is dead?" with "I'm so glad my husband got joy from this." On anniversaries of a loved one's death and on their birthday some people light candles or do balloon releases. I like to ask people to do acts of kindness to keep my husband's smile going.

The more you can recognize the causes of your grief attacks and plan for ways to deal with them, the more you will train your mind to replace moments of agitation with gratitude and/or peace.

Finding Community

Grief is often described as a walk alone, but it can be helpful to find community. Sharing, especially with other grievers, lets us know that what we think is inappropriate or completely strange is normal. However, I also found that being surrounded by grievers all the time added to my sadness. In the first year of my grieving, I decided to take comedy classes. The teacher asked, "Why are you all here?" I said, "My husband died, so I thought I'd do comedy." I learned that community can be found in many places—dancing classes, art classes, a group hike. However, community is not for everyone. If we are isolating, is it because of grief or is it simply because we have always been an introvert?

Day One

"When silentgrief.com quickly grew to a readership in the thousands, I knew there needed to be extra support. So I formed an online Facebook support group: Silent Grief - Child Loss Support. Thousands of bereaved parents and grandparents from around the world now visit daily seeking and receiving help and support."

—CLARA HINTON

Many grief support groups and websites can be found online. One advantage of an online community is that you don't have to leave your house, or even your bed. When you are feeling most stuck, you can turn on your computer and find thousands of people who are also grieving. You may read in silence, or post, or reach out in different ways.

Day Two

"Your community is out there. Look for them. Collect them. Knit them into a vast flotilla of light that can hold you."

—MEGAN DEVINE

After my husband died, I went to a group called Culture Circle. It was a gathering of people who shared poems, songs, stories, paintings, food—any art they had created. It was a warm space I went to once a month. I have never been a group person but as I passed through various groups I met people I have become friends with. My husband used to say, "If you live in your head you live in a very bad neighborhood." I often think that I would be quite comfortable as a hermit, but the truth is, a circle of friends can lift me out of my misery and help me find moments of joy.

Day Three

"That's the nature of grief: It's a creature with many arms but few legs, and it staggers about, searching for support."

—YANN MARTEL

In the first months after my husband's death, I literally staggered all around the world looking for support. I knew I was in trouble. I knew I was saving my own life. I still stagger about, but less so. I have done what I set out to do. I have ever-increasing happy and productive moments. These coexist with my grief.

Day Four

"And it is . . . from the presence of others that we really derive support in our dark hours of grief, and not from their talk, which often only serves to irritate us."

—H. RIDER HAGGARD

Even people who are seeking to comfort can say the most irritating things. In spite of this risk, even the most independent griever can benefit from support. There are people who understand grief and can be present with us in our darkest hours.

Day Five

"I felt as if each person within visual range were slowly draining the life from me. We were all connected, and the more of them there were, the more I wanted to crawl under a table and cry."

—SHAUN DAVID HUTCHINSON

This is the other side. We can crave solitude at the same time as we long for human companionship. I've had the experience of hating being around other people, returning home, and equally hating being alone. There is a balance somewhere. It's different for each person.

Day Six

"Deep grief sometimes is almost like a specific location, a coordinate on a map of time. When you are standing in that forest of sorrow, you cannot imagine that you could ever find your way to a better place. But if someone can assure you that they themselves have stood in that same place, and now have moved on, sometimes this will bring hope."

—ELIZABETH GILBERT

Many people use their grief as a lantern. I share my story and benefit from others who share theirs. You will feel hope again when you are ready. You may already be feeling it and just aren't aware of it yet.

Day Seven

"The great love is gone. There are still little loves— friend to friend, brother to sister, student to teacher. Will you deny yourself comfort at the hearthfire of a cottage because you may no longer sit by the fireplace of a palace? Will you deny yourself to those who reach out to you in hopes of warming themselves at your hearthfire?"

—MERCEDES LACKEY

My great love is gone. Yet over the years I have found comfort at many hearth fires. I do not look to replace or replicate my great love, but I have found other loves. I have also been told that I have quite a warm hearth fire myself. It has become worthwhile to keep it burning so others can warm themselves with me. I will be dead soon enough. While I am alive, I must continually find ways to answer poet Mary Oliver's question: "Tell me, what is it you plan to do with your one wild and precious life?"

Becoming a Grief Whisperer

Make a wish book of things you would like to do, in places where you feel like you might belong. You don't have to do any of them, nor do you have to have the skills to do them. One day, revisit this book and pick one thing to do. Sign up for it. You still don't have to do it. When you are ready, do one thing. If you don't like it, try another. Find the courage to ask someone to have lunch with you or take a walk with you. The worst thing that can happen is that they will say no. I have done more things in my wish book than I ever could have imagined, even in those first months when leaving my bed was so difficult. Impossible things are more possible than we can imagine.

I Don't Like Who I Am Now

Grief can change us in ways we don't particularly like but can't seem to do anything about. The level of stress we live under every day may increase. It is normal to be more grouchy, more sad, more troubled, more tired, more sensitive and simultaneously more insensitive than we have been before. Grief behaves in unexpected ways. We might feel fine one moment and tremendously upset the next. It is common to miss the person we used to be as much as we miss the person who died.

Day One

"Is being a jerk one of the five stages of grief?"

—LISA SCHROEDER

I can be quite temperamental in ways I wasn't before. I often have to apologize to people for snapping at them. I'm so hurt already that any perceived extra dose of hurt has nowhere to go. It overflows in strange ways. The ways in which grief makes us difficult is sometimes what makes it hard for other people to be with us. A grieving person, especially newly grieving, needs patience born out of compassion.

Day Two

"I know that I have lost myself, and I don't know where
to look for her, the strong, funny, capable woman
I used to be . . . I'm a half person, living a half-life,
surrounded by death . . . I hear the long sound coming
before I realize that I am making it, low like a moan.
It is grief, and it is mine."

—ROWAN COLEMAN

I give the appearance of a kind, loving person who accomplishes a lot.
When I leave my house, I often look into the mirror and say, "Please let
me look like a whole person. Please let me sound like a whole person."
I appear to be the same woman I used to be. Yet there is a hollowness
inside me carved out by my grief. I am conscious of all I have achieved.
I am proud of myself. None of it touches the part of me that died when
my husband died.

Day Three

"She couldn't stand how dark and ugly her thoughts
were, how bottomless her anger and grief."

—KRISTIN HANNAH

Grief often manifests itself as anger. Today is the day I am going to be less
angry. Today is the day I am going to be less sad. Then something happens,
and I act in a way I don't like. Maybe I'll change it tomorrow. Maybe I
won't. That's where my apologies come in. There may be an endless
supply of love, but it doesn't stop the constant roiling of anger and grief.

Day Four

"When the worst of the melancholy moments took over me, not even the blue spring sky . . . could remove the darkness inside. Grief was my new companion . . . I hated it, and clung to it at the same time."

—KATIE CROSS

Grievers often cling to their grief. My grief is my love. I walk with it. I hold its hand and it holds mine. Sometimes I hate the way it blinds me to the beauty of the world. Sometimes all I want is a good wallow in it. I am learning to make it a real companion, one that inspires rather than deadens.

Day Five

"But what if the great secret insider-trading truth is that you don't ever get over the biggest losses in your life . . . grief is so frowned upon, so hard for even intimate bystanders to witness that you will think you must be crazy for not getting over it."

—ANNE LAMOTT

It is normal for grievers to feel crazy. Sometimes we feel even crazier because people tell us we are crazy, or stuck or sick. We aren't. Knowing I am not crazy, that others feel like I do, helps me feel less crazy.

Day Six

"I found the adage about time healing all wounds to
be false: grief doesn't fade . . . We are never free from
grief. We are never free from the feeling that we have
failed. We are never free from self-loathing."

—JESMYN WARD

It is normal to internalize the feeling that our culture imposes on us: that
something is wrong with us because we are grieving. We can, if not care-
ful, begin to loathe ourselves for continuing to grieve. The task is not to
stop grieving; the task is to live fully while grieving.

Day Seven

"Great grief can be worn charmingly by a beauty and
I have seen a lot of gracious dignity at funerals in
my time but it's in my experience that when grief is
becoming it is also suspect. Real unhappiness is ugly
and wounding and scarring to the soul."

—JULIAN FELLOWES

Over time I've learned to accept that ugliness, wounding, and scarring
are part of what gives my life meaning. I have given up pretense. I may
acquiesce to others' desire for a quieter, more peaceful side of me when
I am with them, but to know me is to know my hurt. Truly beautiful, truly
charming, are people who have the courage to be real.

Becoming a Grief Whisperer

Sit or lie down in a comfortable place where you will not be interrupted. You can play music or nature sounds. Close your eyes. See if you can feel your loved one holding you or hugging you or touching your face. Remember what it was like to hear their heart beating, the sound of their breathing. Remember when they looked into your eyes and you saw love. Hear their voice. They are saying, "I love you the way you are. Loving you is part of me. I know living without me is difficult and it has changed you. I still love you." You can substitute your own words. Have your loved one say what you want and need to hear.

When you dislike yourself, even for good reasons, it is important to look at yourself not with your own critical eyes, but with the eyes of those who love you and see the good in you that is still there, always there.

Tears

From Biblical to Roman to Victorian times, there have been beautiful bottles made for the purpose of holding tears. Some believe that tears are sacred and have medicinal qualities. Some believe a griever's tears contain different chemicals than regular tears. Some of us cry all the time. Some of us do not cry at all. However much you cry is exactly the right amount.

Day One

"There is a sacredness in tears . . . They are the messengers of overwhelming grief, of deep contrition and of unspeakable love."

—WASHINGTON IRVING

Our grief comes from our love for someone who has died. Our tears are love spilling out of our eyes. It is that unspeakable love turned into overwhelming grief that raises our tears from the profane to the sacred.

Day Two

"The worst type of crying wasn't the kind everyone could see . . . the worst kind happened when your soul wept and no matter what you did, there was no way to comfort it. A section withered and became a scar on the part of your soul that survived."

—KATIE MCGARRY

We have different kinds of crying. One is ragged and comes from deep in our soul. There is nothing for it but to let it tire itself out. Perhaps like water wearing away a stone, that is the way those tears wear away at our souls. There is a scar, but more importantly, there is also survival. Tissue scarring over allows life to continue.

Day Three

"It's so curious: one can resist tears and 'behave' very well in the hardest hours of grief. But then . . . one notices that a flower that was in bud only yesterday has suddenly blossomed, or a letter slips from a drawer . . . and everything collapses."

—COLETTE

Sometimes the simplest gesture triggers the collapse into tears of sorrow. We carry our grief with us wherever we go, and many days it's easily hidden. Then something reflects our loss in such a way that our eyes become like waterfalls. I have found that as years go by, these moments happen less and less, and only rarely in public.

Day Four

"American men are allotted just as many tears as American women. But because we are forbidden to shed them, we die long before women do, with our hearts exploding or our blood pressure rising or our livers eaten away by alcohol because that lake of grief inside us has no outlet. We, men, die because our faces were not watered enough."

—PAT CONROY

The grief of men is as sharp and deep as that of women. I was glad that my husband felt free to cry when he was mourning the death of his best friend. Many people, including health professionals and researchers, believe that the failure to express emotion can lead to physical problems, even death.

Day Five

"Tears aren't for the people we've lost. They're for us. So we can remember, and celebrate, and miss them, and feel human."

C.J. REDWINE

This speaks to the essential and acceptable selfishness of grief. Those who have died are most likely fine. Our tears are for our own pain of missing; they are also a celebration of our love. We cry because we are human and we are left behind here on Earth.

Day Six

"I cry a lot because I miss people. They die and I can't stop them. They leave me and I love them more."

—MAURICE SENDAK

Maybe it is okay to accept frequent crying as the natural expression of missing people and our powerlessness over death. Many people don't understand that love continues to grow even after death.

Day Seven

"Tears are a river that takes you somewhere . . . Tears lift your boat off the rocks, off dry ground, carrying it downriver to someplace better."

—CLARISSA PINKOLA ESTÉS

I often think of tears as a symptom of being stuck. What if instead, they are a symbol of movement? The more I cry, the more I move on. With crying, we are taken to a place that is better. What does your better place look or feel like? Is it some place you are ready to find?

Becoming a Grief Whisperer

Keep a tears journal for at least a week. Before you go to sleep, write down how often you cried and for how long. If you didn't cry at all, note that. Give your tears a voice, and write what they are saying. If you haven't cried, write down what your uncried tears want to tell you. Now, lie down, close your eyes, and picture how light refracting through raindrops creates a beautiful rainbow. Picture light refracting through your tears, real or imaginary, creating a beautiful rainbow of love that reaches from you to your loved one. Use this rainbow connection to fall off into sleep, filled with this sense of loving connection. This is the better place your tears are taking you to.

Considering Suicide

When my husband died, I expected him to come back and get me. When he didn't, I thought it was my responsibility to go to him. I researched suicide. In the end, I could not give the grief that had been given to me to others. I could not give my daughter the lifelong pain of a mother's suicide. I couldn't give pain to anyone who might find my lifeless body. Having reluctantly decided to live, I had to figure out how. That's where my journey began, and why it continues to this day. There is nothing wrong with considering suicide, but it is so much braver to choose life. I still want to be with my husband, but I am willing to wait. When I look back on the past eight years, there is so much I would have missed. I am alive because I am supposed to be alive. I am not always happy being alive, but I am happy that I chose life. I will be with my husband soon enough.

If you need someone to talk to, please call the National Suicide Prevention Lifeline at 1-800-273-TALK (8255). If you get someone you don't like talking to, hang up and call at a different time when different people will be there. It is free to call and open 24 hours a day.

Day One

"Why? Why was it that in cases of real love the one
who is left does not more often follow the beloved by
suicide . . . Or perhaps, when there is love, (we) must
stay for the resurrection of the beloved—so that the
one who has gone is not really dead, but grows and is
created for a second time in the soul of the living?"

—CARSON MCCULLERS

When someone we love dies, we may not feel we can survive the pain of
another breath. What greater comfort could there be than joining them?
Yet perhaps there is a reason for our continued life. Part of grief work is
discovering this reason. I do know that the following is true: No one can
keep our loved ones alive and remembered better than we can.

Day Two

"The thought of suicide is a great consolation: by
means of it one gets through many a dark night."

—FRIEDRICH NIETZSCHE

The thought of suicide is different than the act of suicide. It is possible to
use thinking of our own death as a comfort, while at the same time knowing that this is thought only. We can speed along our wish to be reunited
with those we love in our imagination, while continuing to do the daily
work that leads us to being fully alive with grief.

Day Three

"Killing yourself slowly is still killing yourself. Wanting to die is not the same as wanting to come home. Recovery is hard work. Not wanting to die is hard work."

—BLYTHE BAIRD

One of the most important parts of grief work is moving from wanting to die to wanting to live, to come home to oneself, however different that self is now. I have known more than one griever who made suicidal gestures and thought happiness was beyond reach. In time, these same grievers returned to the living. They miss their loved ones still, and yet their lives are deep and rich and wanted. When we can't yet see the path, it may still be there.

Day Four

"[He] wondered, and not for the first time . . . if this was the day that missing her would finally be too much for him."

—DENNIS LEHANE

We miss our loved ones so intensely that we sometimes project ourselves into a future where the unbearable pain of missing them will finally be too much. If that day comes, we think we will have to stop this pain any way we can. We can also wonder if this will be the day that we can begin to honor their life by making our own life full again.

Day Five

"Grief is one big, gaping hole, isn't it . . . It's everywhere and all consuming. Some days you think you can't go on because the only thing waiting for you is more despair."

—MARIEKE NIJKAMP

Living with grief takes moment-to-moment courage. It is often described as a black hole that we are thrown into with no way to climb out. The despair seems endless. It makes us feel that going on is useless. Yet we do go on. We need to not only feel the moments where something besides despair is in our hearts and minds, we also need to notice that we are feeling them. We find that grief is everywhere, but so is love.

Day Six

"The word 'survivor' . . . carries a weight of remembrance that has broken the minds and bodies of more than a few . . . It also . . . compels many to do whatever they can to help reinforce the efforts of those who might be 'at risk' of not just giving up on their dreams, but of giving up on their continued existence."

—ABERJHANI

Remembrance should be joy, but it can also be a weight. We wonder why and how we have survived. When our future has been shattered, how do we still make our dreams come true? One way is to hold hands and hearts with those who are considering giving up their existence. Together we hold each other up.

Day Seven

"The bravest thing I ever did was continuing my life when I wanted to die."

—JULIETTE LEWIS

If we can be brave enough to keep breathing, to keep living when all we want is to be with those who have gone before us, we have the hope of becoming fully alive with grief. I hold my husband's hand as he pulls me forward because I want to make him proud.

Becoming a Grief Whisperer

Write a commitment to life contract. Start with, "I promise to stay alive for six months." Then write at least 10 reasons why you will stay alive. Include your unwillingness to pass your grief on to others. Think of people, pets, and things you love. You can include things that you used to love. Write down things that your loved one would want you to do. Write down three actions you will take. These could include calling a suicide hotline (1-800-273-8255), seeing a grief counselor, taking a class in meditation or yoga, or hiking. If you have trouble moving, simple actions like taking a shower or looking at comics or lovely pictures on the Internet will do.

When the six months have ended, if you need to, you can renew the contract. This is not only a contract with yourself; it is also a contract with the person you love that died.

WEEK 29
Despair

Despair is one of grief's most potent weapons. As long as we are alive there is hope for us, but grief often blots it out. In a total solar eclipse, the sun does not go away, it is only hidden behind the shadow cast upon it. In the total eclipse of hope, hope is merely hidden behind the shadow cast by grief.

Day One

> "How does one even begin to pull oneself out of such deep despair? No footholds, nothing to grab onto . . . You ask yourself, do I even want to? Perhaps I will stay in this place of darkness forever."
>
> —DONNA VISOCKY

There is something comfortable about despair. We can sink into the abyss and lie still in darkness forever. We can be dead while we are still alive. Or we can close our eyes and imagine a hard climb out. We can even imagine a trampoline that will bounce us out, when we are ready.

Day Two

"Despair can come from deep grief, but it can also be a defense against the risks of bitter disappointment and shattering heartbreak . . . To choose hope is to step firmly forward into the howling wind, baring one's chest to the elements, knowing that, in time, the storm will pass."

—DESMOND TUTU

Who, in a safe place of isolation and womb-like darkness, wishes to walk out into the howling wind of the violent storms of grief? We do. That is why we seek help. We are grief warriors, and our grief requires us to be fiercer than we have ever been. Even if the storm has blown our world to bits, we will find a way to rebuild.

Day Three

"She wondered that hope was so much harder than despair."

—PATRICIA BRIGGS

Is hope harder or easier than despair? Part of grief work is hearing the quiet call of hope through the deafening shriek of despair.

Day Four

"The saddest kind of blues is for them that's had everything they ever wanted and has lost it, and knows it won't come back no more. Ain't no sufferin' in this world worse than that; and that's the blues we call 'I Had It But It's All Gone Now.'"

—KEN GRIMWOOD

The saddest kind of blues is for those of us who live knowing a loved one who died can't come back. We want them to come back; we plead for them, sometimes we even think we see them or hear them, that they have come back. It's being lucky enough to have had something precious to lose, and being unlucky enough to live every day with the loss.

Day Five

"Missing someone is the worst form of torture because it never goes away . . . And no matter how much times passes, you still feel the ache of their absence whenever they rise into your thoughts."

—CAROLINE GEORGE

This is the center of despair. Our desperate missing will always be a part of us. This is the secret most of us learn not to speak. Time does not soften the torture of the ache of the absence of the person we love. We are prisoners of war who learn to survive and even thrive.

Day Six

"How the coming of the dusk dissolves the laces of the splint that holds you together during the day, and the . . . heaviness of opening your eyes the next morning when you realize that you've begun another day of grief . . . "

—HOPE JAHREN

Despair is part of who I am now. During the day there are things to do, which sometimes holds me together. Then I come home to my loneliness and look for the solace of sleep, hoping for escape rather than insomnia or nightmare. Then I awake and remember and find the courage to do it all over again. I do not want to be fixed because I cannot be fixed. However, I can accomplish more broken than I ever imagined I could in those first days of chaos and complete despair.

Day Seven

"I remember thinking, 'How does anyone survive something like this? And if they do, what kind of person comes out the other end?' I didn't know, but throughout that dark time of grief, sorrow, desolation, and complete despair, something in me seemed determined to carry on."

—NEIL PEART

What is the thing in us that stirs up the life force? What is the thing in us that is determined to carry on? Is it that we were/are loved? Is it that we don't want to disappoint those who have loved us? I believe my husband holds me gently when I am in the deepest throes of despair, and I believe he smiles in whatever way the dead smile when he sees me happy. When he was alive he admired how every time I fell down I found a way to stand up again. Now I must let his admiration and love pull me back up when I have fallen down.

Becoming a Grief Whisperer

Picture your despair as a storm cloud, dark and heavy, that you hold in your cupped hands. Put everything that defines your despair into that cloud. Now blow it away. Search all of your being for despair, and continue to breathe it out into as many storm clouds as you need. Each time the darkness reassembles, blow it away. Now imagine how it looks when just one ray of sun peeks through the clouds after the storm. What is that ray of sunshine? Is it something your loved one said? Is it someone living who is still precious to you? Is it a painting or a brightly colored flower? When you are ready, add as many rays of sunshine to this exercise as you wish. Feel their warmth, on you and within you.

Hope

Hope is the life force trying to come through. Hope is seeing stars brighten the dark night. It's knowing that sunset is followed by sunrise. It may feel like grief kills all hope, but hope has a way of waiting for us to be ready to rediscover it.

Day One

"The journey across the landscape of loss to the inner self takes courage and persistence. It is a risky venture, with lots of false trails and humanizing errors . . . But . . . it is a journey on which there is always hope."

—DR. BRIAN BABINGTON

It is possible to make ourselves understand that there is always hope. It may be hidden and require courage and persistence to uncover, but that does not mean it is not there. Language is important. If we say, "I will find hope," we allow for the possibility of this happening, even when it seems impossible.

Day Two

"My childhood ended the day my brother died. The naive hope that a miracle would save him, that he would one day walk, that a disease was a blessing in my family—that hope died with him."

—DARCY LEECH

We often feel that hope dies along with the person we love. Our hopes for our future are irrevocably changed. Our hopes for the person to fight, to live, to survive, are gone. If we can no longer pray with hope, we can pray for hope. If we prefer not to pray, we can visualize.

Day Three

"A flood of emotions rushes into me. Pain and anger. Sadness and pity. But most surprising of all, hope."

—JAY ASHER

Like a cool breeze on a hot summer day, we can be in the midst of our grief and feel the soft touch of hope on our cheek, hear the soft whisper of hope in our ear. The underground spring that nourishes hope is love.

Day Four

"Don't try to find a sunbeam where a shroud of darkness encloses me. Let me mourn. Then, after the storm, when the tears have run dry and my eyes choose to open, I will look for your rainbow of hope."

—RICHELLE E. GOODRICH

There is a certain timing for the message of hope to reach us. To force ourselves to consider hope too early can make us cynical about the possibility of it appearing. It is often best to sit in our anguish and allow our tears to flow. Hope will come when you are ready, not before.

Day Five

"Hope is the feeling we have that the feeling we have is not permanent."

—MIGNON MCLAUGHLIN

Grief may be permanent, but the shape and weight and size of it are not. At first, its presence may be all that there is. Hopefully in time, we will become fully alive with grief. In time, we will be grieving while fully alive with hope.

Day Six

"Hope rises like a phoenix from the ashes of shattered dreams."

—S.A. SACHS

How can the mythical phoenix rise from its ashes? We don't need to know how. We only need to know that it does. When our loved ones die it can seem as though we only have the ashes of our shattered dreams. I have found hope rising in the most unexpected ways in the most unexpected places.

Day Seven

"Hope is not logical. It always comes as a surprise, just when you think all hope is lost. Hope is the cousin to grief, and both take time: you can't short-circuit grief, or emptiness, and you can't patch it up . . . You have to take the next right action."

—ANNE LAMOTT

Just as we were surprised by the intensity of grief, we may be surprised by the vibrancy of hope. If hope is cousin to grief, perhaps it is just waiting to be invited to the family gathering. With confusion being one of the weapons of grief, how do we pause to let the clarity of the next right action appear to us? Perhaps it already has.

Becoming a Grief Whisperer

Buy enough black marbles or black glass gems (available in craft stores or online) to fill a bowl or jar. Buy a few colored marbles or glass gems. If you prefer, you can substitute faith/wishing stones or minerals.

Fill your container with the black marbles or gems. Then place one colored marble, gem, or stone in with the black. Close your eyes and mix them around. Now open your eyes and find the colored one. Take it out. This is your hope. Hold it in your hands. Put it next to your heart. What does hope feel like to you? What does finding hope mean to you?

When you are ready, put in two colored pieces among the black ones. Now hope is a little easier to find. Increase the number of colored pieces as much as you want. The darkness of your grief can make room for color, light, and hope. Write about this experience if you wish. You may take your piece of hope with you so it is available for you to touch or hold at any time.

So Much Left Unsaid, So Much Left Undone

No one ever dies at the right time. There are always things we wish we had said or done. Even if we did our very best, as days pass we experience new things we want to say and do. Part of the recurring trauma of grief is the inability to share our lives with the person we love. The only thing that would genuinely help is for our loved ones to be alive again, and that is the one thing we cannot have.

Day One

"The bitterest tears shed over graves are for words left unsaid and deeds left undone."

—HARRIET BEECHER STOWE

I think of all the time we wasted. We had many loving moments, but we could have had so many more. All those hours in our separate rooms, thinking what we were doing was more important than being together, until being together was no longer possible. I want those moments back.

Day Two

"All of life like a series of tableaux, and in the living we missed so much, hid so much, left so much undone and unsaid."

—ANNA QUINDLEN

It is a normal part of grieving to go back over every moment and think about how we could have done it differently if only we were more aware our time was limited. When people are alive, it is easy to take the future for granted. Then someone dies and our priorities shift, but there is nothing we can do to change things now.

Day Three

"A relationship between two people is made up . . . of invisible things: memories, shared experiences, hopes and fears . . . Memories can do a lot to sustain you, but the invisible stuff of the relationship is lost, even as unresolved issues remain: arguments never settled, kind words never uttered, things left unsaid . . . "

—DAVID DOSA

No one can ever take the place of the one we love. We understand each other in so many unique ways, with shared history, shared memories, shared emotions that will never be repeated. There are things that cannot be resolved, and kindnesses of thought and gesture that cannot be directly expressed. We do not have to have this in the forefront of our mind for it to be a constant source of hurt.

Day Four

"I'm never going to see him again. There were so many things I didn't say, and after my parents . . . I swore I'd never leave anything unsaid. But I did. Now he's gone."

—MYRA MCENTIRE

After my husband died, I knew it was important to say things before people died. I planned to call a friend who had cancer, but she died before I made the call. The only thing I could do was picture her smiling face and know that she would have forgiven me. Because she would forgive me, I forgive myself.

Day Five

"The worst part about losing someone you love— besides the agony of never getting to see them again—are the things you never said. The unsaid stalks you, mocks you for thinking you had all the time in the world."

—KAREN MARIE MONING

I want to tell you I'm sorry for not understanding you better. I want to tell you I am sorry for not spending more time with you. I thought we had forever. I knew you were dying. I just didn't expect you to die that moment, that day. Maybe that's why I still talk to you. I want to make it right by believing you can still hear me.

Day Six

"If only time had allowed me to understand the things I would want to say after you were gone. That's the thing. They told me 'don't leave anything unsaid.' But I didn't know what I wanted to say until it was too late . . . "

—JACQUELINE SIMON GUNN

I understand you so much better now than I did when you were alive. On the eighth anniversary of your death, I watched a video of you. I laughed because it took me that long to understand, in a new way, the gifts you gave me every day. I thought I had said everything. I did say the most important thing, that I love you.

Day Seven

"I'm sorry for all the ways I failed you."
"I am too."

—ARTHUR AND JAN WARNER

I was lucky to spend my husband's dying time with him. He was a proud peacock of a man. When he looked at me and said, "I'm sorry for all the ways I failed you," it was as though everything was stripped away and we were back in the pure flowering of our love. My response was simple, "I am too." The truth is that no matter how long we have someone with us, it is never long enough. There will always be things left unsaid, things left undone.

Becoming a Grief Whisperer

Write your loved one a letter. Tell them all the things you want to say. Write as many letters as you wish. If you prefer not to write, picture their beloved face before you. Look into their remembered eyes. Talk to them. Tell them everything. Listen for their response. If you don't hear anything, imagine what they would say.

WEEK 32

Regret

I try not to regret things in the past because I cannot change
them. Yet the regret comes anyway. My antidote to regret
is to think on the things that I did do, instead of the things I
failed to do.

Day One

"There seemed to be no easy correlation between the
awful grief I felt at her death and our closeness—or
lack of it—in life, and it occurred to me that perhaps
grief is as much regret for what we have never had as
sorrow for what we have lost."

—DAVID NICHOLLS

We grieve for what we have lost. We grieve also for what we never had.
The ways in which we could have shared more, done more, expressed our
love better. There is no opportunity now to make it better. It will always be
what it was. This is especially difficult when someone dies with whom we
had a difficult relationship or hadn't seen or spoken to for a long time.

Day Two

"Grief was something you could work through, but
regret lived forever, tormenting you with everything
you might have done differently."

—KIT ROCHA

Regret seems to live forever because the ability to do things differently is
gone. I want to go back and change things. I can't. I want to go forward and
change things. I can change things in myself, but not in my relationship to
my loved one who has died.

Day Three

"Nothing crushes the soul of a father more than the loss of the beloved son he failed to lavish his love on."

—JANVIER CHOUTEU-CHANDO

This is true for all relationships. How, we wonder, could we have shown our love more completely? Why did we think other things were more important than actively showing our love for each other?

Day Four

"People really could be one way outside, when inside they were torn to shreds, a fine white powder of grief and regret replacing blood and bones, and no one even noticed."

—ALICE HOFFMAN

Regret, like grief, often remains hidden. We present a smiling face to the world and no one sees behind our facade. Regret and grief. Why do you not notice?

Day Five

"Grief and sorrow are one and the same. But until you feel regret for what is now forever out of reach, you do not truly mourn."

—CAMERON DOKEY

Is regret an essential component of mourning? Perhaps for a time. I would rather replace regret with self-compassion and memory of love. When I am ready.

Day Six

"R-E-G-R-E-T. I can spell that word now. Raw. Endless. Grief. Raining. Eternal. Tears."

—KAREN MARIE MONING

There is regret for all that is lost. There is regret for grieving. There is regret for regret. The raining of tears that seems endless.

Day Seven

"When we regret that we don't have more memories of them . . . gradually we find ourselves remembering them being with us in times and places that they couldn't have been, and gradually we stop correcting ourselves because, well, we want them to have been there."

—DATHAN AUERBACH

It is devastating to acknowledge that no new memories can be created with the ones we love so much. Our earthly time with them has ended. There is sometimes a fear that we will forget things. We wonder if something really happened a certain way or if we are inventing it. Maybe that doesn't matter. Reality is, after all, subjective.

Becoming a Grief Whisperer

On small pieces of paper, write things that you regret not saying or doing. When you have finished, gather the pieces of paper and burn them in an ashtray or fireplace. If you don't have a safe place to burn them, put them in an envelope and throw the envelope away. Write a letter to your loved one telling them all the things you wish you had said and done. Ask them to forgive you. Put this letter in an envelope and keep it for a while. You can open it at a later date and add more thoughts, if you need to. When you are finished, quietly ask yourself for forgiveness. You may be able to forgive yourself in this moment, or if not, when you are ready.

I've Lost My Way

When someone who is central to our life dies, it is normal to feel that we have lost our way, and our path in life has been ripped away. Nothing prepares us for the reality of death. Our own life feels like it has stopped. We need to resuscitate ourselves and create new meaning for our lives.

Day One

> "He always thought that (her) long illness would somehow prepare him for her death. He always imagined that grief and guilt . . . would be more clear-edged, more defined, more finite."
>
> —JULIAN BARNES

No matter how long someone is ill, or how old they are, we are never prepared for their death. We are often startled by the infinite, hard to grasp nature of both our grief and our guilt.

Day Two

"It is not a 'healing journey.' It's a 'numb slog' . . . if they call it a 'healing journey,' it's just a day of you eating Wheat Thins for breakfast in your underwear, you're like 'I guess I'm f–king up my healing journey.' But if they would say you're going to have a 'numb slog,' you could say 'oh, I'm nailing it.'"

—PATTON OSWALT

If people were more honest about the true nature of grieving, we wouldn't feel we were somehow doing it wrong. I call it grief work because it is work. It's not a healing journey, like we get to go on a cruise to somewhere full of sunshine. If we stay in bed today, if we plan to do something and find we can't today, if we are lost again in a swirl of emotions we can't control today, we are "nailing it." We are always exactly where we are supposed to be at any given time. Sometimes just continuing to breathe is enough.

Day Three

"What is it like when you lose someone you love?" Jane asked.
"You die, too. And you wait around for your body to catch up."

—JOHN SCALZI

I call it "decorating the waiting room." I thought I died when my husband did, and I would continue my life as an empty shell. Part of me is still just waiting to be with him in the same form. Yet grief work is learning that while we are still alive, we can fill our lives with joy and purpose. We can manage to die and live at the same time.

Day Four

"When we lose people we love, we don't mourn the past—we mourn un-lived tomorrows. We mourn the loss of people who knew us thoroughly and loved us anyway, and future memories that will never be made."

—JAMES RUSSELL LINGERFELT

We often feel lost because the person who showed us how to find our way has died. All our future plans are gone, and we cannot imagine how we will come up with new ones. We sometimes cannot imagine why we would even want to.

Day Five

"Some people appear to thrive after trauma. Loss emboldens them . . . I couldn't find it in me to do much more than reel from one day and year to the next, with little optimism about what lay ahead . . . "

—CATRIONA MENZIES-PIKE

As many resources as there are, at times none of them seem to help. It can feel like permanent vertigo as we reel forward in time, never quite finding a way to steady ourselves. Are others thriving, or do they feel like I do but keep their true feelings hidden?

Day Six

"Your identity is altered, even though you don't want it to be. You are not the same person, and some of your friends will relate to you differently. Redefining ourselves, that is, building a new identity after the death of a loved one, is another significant task commonly forgotten in grief work."

—LOUIS E. LAGRAND

After someone who is central to our life dies, we are different. Other people wait, sometimes impatiently, for us to return to who we were. We can learn to rebuild, much as someone who comes home after a hurricane to find their home is destroyed can build a new home, but if we hope to be the same as before, we may be disappointed. It is helpful to me to know that this happens to many people—it didn't just happen to me.

Day Seven

"Perhaps," said the man, "you would like to be lost with us. I have found it much more agreeable to be lost in the company of others."

—KATE DICAMILLO

The loss of someone we love is never a good thing, but the loss of ourselves might be. It might be an opportunity to become someone new and turn all our ideas of feeling lost upside down. Let's not do this alone. We can have an "I'm lost, too" party just to see what happens next.

Becoming a Grief Whisperer

Without making a plan, walk, drive, or take public transportation to a place you have never been before. (Do this only in safe places.) Take a bus and get off at a random stop. Walk and turn left when you have always turned right. Drive along roads you have never been on before. See what you pass along the way and where you end up. Now, find your way back. No technology—just use your memory and your own sense of place. If you are nervous about getting too lost, have your GPS or a map close at hand. Sometimes being lost can be an adventure.

Afterlife

Everyone we love who dies has an afterlife. It may be a continuation of consciousness in some form. It may be in the stories we continue to tell and the love we still feel. Soon after my husband died, a man who worked at the UPS store insistently offered to carry my boxes to my car. He knew us only as occasional customers. When we reached my car, he said, "Your husband came to me and said I had to tell you that you have to know how much he loves you." I laughed, saying, "That must have been a heck of a dream." His seriousness intensified. "It wasn't a dream. It was an apparition. You must always know how much your husband loves you." Tears fell from my eyes. Now I ask people, "What does UPS deliver to you?"

Day One

"If I die, I will wait for you, do you understand? No matter how long. I will watch from beyond to make sure you live every year you have to its fullest, and then we'll have so much to talk about when I see you again."

—JEANIENE FROST

Something that can motivate us is the thought of sharing things with the ones we love when we are reunited with them. When it is my time, and I am asked what I have done, I don't want my answer to be, "Not much." Even if I didn't believe my husband was waiting for me, it still motivates me to think I am doing things he would be proud of.

Day Two

"We see a hearse; we think sorrow. We see a grave; we think despair. We hear of a death; we think of a loss. Not so in heaven. When heaven sees a breathless body, it sees the vacated cocoon & the liberated butterfly."

—MAX LUCADO

It was only as I sat with my husband's dead body that I understood why they called this empty vessel "the remains." It is my loss but I sincerely hope it is his gain. How powerful must his spirit be, freed from his ailing and aged body. Fly free, my love. Fly free.

Day Three

"The bird is gone, and in what meadow does it now sing?"

—PHILIP K. DICK

Some people have a definite idea of what the afterlife is. In our family, we call it "The Great Unknown." If there is consciousness after death—and I believe there is—I hope our loved ones are singing their song even more brightly than when they were alive.

Day Four

"I promise to love you forever in this life and wherever we go in the afterlife, because I know I can't go on in any life unless you're in it too."

—J.A. REDMERSKI

We were connected before we met and continue to be connected. When we love someone deeply, it's common to have a sense of familiarity that is beyond logic, even if they are no longer present physically. That sense of continued connection can be a great comfort.

Day Five

"I imagine how good it must feel to them to know how much they are still loved and missed in this realm, and for a moment I let myself feel them loving me back."

—CLAIRE BIDWELL SMITH

Does love remain an eternal circle after death? I hope my loved ones know how much I love and miss them. When I am quiet, I can feel them loving me back. My grief gentles down when I remain in the center of the eternal circle of love.

Day Six

"The tragedy was that we knew we would never
see each other again . . . I don't think I'll ever
see Carl again. But I saw him. We saw each other.
We found each other in the cosmos, and that
was wonderful."

—ANN DRUYAN

You don't have to believe in an afterlife to find comfort in love. Our loved
ones live on in our heart and in our memory. Carl Sagan and Ann Druyan
did not believe they'd see each other after death, but they were still filled
with the joy of the time they spent together here on Earth.

Day Seven

"From grief over the warm and ardent love which she
had lost and still secretly mourned . . . Through the
great darkness that would come, she saw the gleam
of another, gentler sun, and she sensed the fragrance
of the herbs in the garden at world's end."

—SIGRID UNDSET

Sometimes the veil between this life on Earth and the life that comes after
thins, and we get a sense of the warmth and sweetness to come. What connects the two realms? Love.

Becoming a Grief Whisperer

Let your loved ones who have died gather around you and tell you stories about where they are now. Ask questions and see if they will answer. If you don't hear or see them, use your imagination. You can do this as a quiet meditation with your eyes closed. You can write it as a poem or story. You can illustrate it. If you feel it is not possible, or unwise, to talk with the dead, have your beloved dead gather around you in your memory and share moments of when they were alive that you are grateful for. Acknowledge how alive they are in you as you tell their stories.

Love

There are no words strong or poetic enough to define love. We know in our own hearts what our love is and continues to be. To have someone return our love creates a never-ending circle that is one of the most precious things we have in life: a blessing and a gift. It is my belief that love triumphs over and transcends death. If you believe in an afterlife, the love continues as a vibrant circle. If you don't believe in an afterlife, the love still continues as a vibrant feeling in your heart, mind, and soul.

Day One

"Grief is tremendous, but love is bigger. You are grieving because you loved truly. The beauty in that is greater than the bitterness of death. Allowing this into your consciousness will not keep you from suffering, but it will help you survive the next day."

—CHERYL STRAYED

Acknowledge grief, but remember love. Grief can break us into pieces, while love is the glue that puts us back together. Hopefully at some point, love will allow grief to inspire you rather than deaden you, but if nothing else, it can give you the strength to survive the next minute, the next hour, the next day.

Day Two

"I don't think grief is a price we pay for love, but rather that it is a part of love. When death comes, I think the grief is to be experienced the way the joy was experienced before—and if we experience it intimately, grief and joy are not separate, and both are love."

—BARRY GRAHAM

It took me several years to realize that grief was also joy, because it was the result of my experiencing love. How much more tragic would it have been to be married and not grieve for my husband? If we start noticing the love in our grief, perhaps we can start to notice the joy in our grief—the joy of love.

Day Three

"But in all of the sadness . . . You've got to remember that grief isn't the absence of love. Grief is the proof that love is still there."

—TESSA SHAFFER

Grief empties us of everything we value in ourselves. What if that emptiness is actually a fullness? What if the hole is filled with love? Love doesn't take away the pain and the ache of missing, but it helps us hold it in a different way.

Day Four

"We may bury their bodies or scatter their ashes, but their spirits are boundless and do not accompany them to the grave. Instead of insisting on figuratively burying our dead, why not keep them close to us? Love doesn't die when we do."

—APRIL SLAUGHTER

It is a misconception that in order to "heal" or "find acceptance" we have to let go of our beloved dead. If we hold on we are accused of "living in the past" or "being stuck." The past informs our present. Forgetting the past is amnesia. It is foolish to not remember a love that keeps us whole. Our connection with our loved ones can remain strong in a healthy way if we allow it.

Day Five

"When you love someone, they're always waiting for you. Love transcends everything—even death."

—AMANDA M. LEE

I believe that my loved ones are waiting for me, but even if they are not, I still believe our love is transcendent. You can't see electricity, but you can harness it and use it to create light. You can't see love, but if you believe it continues to exist, you can harness it and use it to fuel the inner light of your spirit.

Day Six

"I believe that imagination is stronger than knowledge. That myth is more potent than history. That dreams are more powerful than facts. That hope always triumphs over experience. That laughter is the only cure for grief. And I believe that love is stronger than death."

—ROBERT FULGHUM

Love is stronger than death. Just as we exercise our physical muscles to make our bodies stronger, we can exercise our emotional love and memory of love muscles to make our spirit stronger.

Day Seven

"Though lovers be lost, love shall not; And death shall have no dominion."

—DYLAN THOMAS

I am cynical about a lot of things, but I truly believe that love outwits death. Love triumphs over death. Death consumes the body but has no dominion over the power of love.

Becoming a Grief Whisperer

Buy a pad of sticky notes. Each morning when you wake up, and each night before you go to sleep, write one thing about the love you share with the person who has died. It could be something you did together. It can be specific, like "I love how we used to laugh at bad puns" or a feeling, like "I love you." You can put the notes in your journal or stick them anywhere—on your bathroom mirror, the refrigerator, walls, in your car—so your environment is filled with reminders of love.

Crazy Things Grievers Do

When someone we love dies, we do things that seem crazy to others or ourselves. It's our attempt to do anything we can think of to keep our connection with our loved one and to bring some small measure of comfort to ourselves. Whatever you are doing, if it isn't hurting you or anyone else, it's okay, and I promise you many other people are doing exactly the same thing.

Day One

"When I wear her clothes, I just feel safer, like she's whispering in my ear."

—JANDY NELSON

I still wear my husband's shirts to sleep in. They've been washed many times and don't have any of his DNA left on them, but I still wear them. I also have a jacket of his that I often wear—it feels like he is hugging me. Sometimes I feel a bit silly but I'm not. This is normal. I'm grieving.

Day Two

"I'll never throw these small things away. There will never be a time when I don't want them, all the tiny parts of Cal that made a life."

—CATH CROWLEY

Grievers often can't decide whether to give things away, and if they do, when is the appropriate time. The appropriate time is when it feels right. Some people keep everything forever. They are part of our loved one's life and therefore part of them. I didn't have room for my husband's drums in my new apartment, so I gave them to someone who loves him, too. On certain days I tell our friend, "Bang those drums!"

Day Three

"I pulled a dirty black sweatshirt from the laundry basket on my son's floor and tried to drink in his scent, to savor the essence of my sweet boy. I inhaled it long and hard, wanting to permanently implant all of him in my brain, to make him last forever."

—SHELLEY RAMSEY

We wish we could bury ourselves in the scent of our loved one. Maybe that's why there is a reluctance to wash their things. Eventually their scent disappears. If only we could keep all of them with us.

Day Four

"She does not want to feel even the faintest temptation
to call his mobile number, as she had done obsessively
for the first year after his death so she could hear
his voice on the answering service . . . But today,
the Anniversary of the day he died, is a day when all
bets are off."

—JOJO MOYES

How many of us have called our loved one's phone number or texted
them? When my husband first died, I listened to his voice mails to see if
I had missed notifying someone. One day I heard a woman sobbing and
wondered who it was. It was me. I used to leave him messages. I knew
he couldn't get them, but it made him feel less dead to do that. It is quite
common to repeat old familiar grief behaviors on anniversaries and other
difficult dates.

Day Five

"I don't guffaw at the woman who visits her husband's
grave and chats him up every now and then, maybe
on the anniversary of his death . . . if I have difficul-
ties with the ontological status of who she's talking to,
that's all right. That's not what this is about. This is
about humans being human."

—CARL SAGAN

Carl Sagan, the renowned scientist and atheist, believed there was no one
there to talk to after a death. He still retained his compassion for the need
of survivors for continued communication with their beloved dead. It is
simply part of our being human.

Day Six

> "Sometimes, even after someone dies, you want to send them a postcard."
>
> —DR. SUNWOLF

Sometimes we send our loved ones who have died a postcard or a letter, or do a balloon release. The desire to keep our connection alive in any way we can does not end with death. A common postcard sentiment is our strongest desire: "Wish you were here."

Day Seven

> "I'm a 5'2 woman totally unwilling to let go of the 6'1 man's tweed suit from circa 1950 that's hanging in my closet ... Fortunately ... when it comes to grief, crazy is the new normal."
>
> —ELEANOR HALEY

Crazy is normal if we celebrate our differences and allow for freedom of expression. The "crazy" things that grievers do are not pathological. They are a natural part of who we have become.

Becoming a Grief Whisperer

What would you like to do but you haven't done it because it seems crazy? Would you like to buy a dead loved one a present, call their number, or wear their clothes? Either take the action or imagine taking the action. Write a few words about how you feel.

Is there something you do that you would like to stop doing? Stop doing it for as long as feels comfortable. Write a few words about how you feel.

If you decide to give things away but are uncertain of how you will handle it afterward, give them to a friend or somewhere that you can get them back. Keeping things is okay. Changing what you decide to keep is also okay.

Keep playing with what are the actions you can give yourself permission to do to bring you comfort and the actions you no longer need.

Those Dates: Anniversaries, Birthdays, Holidays

Feelings of grief often intensify around various dates that were celebratory when our loved ones were still alive. Other people are in a festive mode; stores and e-mail boxes are crammed with happy, while we are sad or angry. We have one extra date on our calendar: the anniversary of our loved one's death. I have had some success at returning some dates back to their original joyous state, but not all of them and not all the time.

Day One

"How can you celebrate togetherness when there is none? When you have lost someone special, your world loses its celebratory qualities. Holidays only magnify the loss. The sadness feels sadder and the loneliness goes deeper."

—ELISABETH KÜBLER-ROSS

Holidays may stop being joyous. They may magnify loss and pain. If we sit at a holiday table, all we may see is the absence of the person we love. The sadness and loneliness are greater when the entire world is holding hands and ours are empty of the hand we want to be holding.

Day Two

"Are you ok? they'll say. Tomorrow is the one-year anniversary of my dad's death, and since he's still dead, I am not okay."

—LOLA ST. VIL

No. I'm not okay. But it's okay not to be okay. It's okay to say that since the one we love is still dead and will always be dead, the question "Are you okay?" is not for us. It is meant for others to find comfort, and sometimes we lie to give them that comfort.

Day Three

"I thought I was long done with the Firsts. First Easter since his death, First Birthday, First Trip to IHOP, First Phillies Game. But everything . . . that we'd never share again . . . still waited before me. In that moment, I dreaded the rest of my life."

—JERI SMITH-READY

Some people say grieving doesn't get easier with time; it gets harder. We have to get through the firsts, then the seconds, then the thirds, and on and on. It can make us dread the rest of our lives. Then we can remember how we were loved, and perhaps in between the dreadful moments we can have some wonderful moments.

Day Four

"There are moments amidst their celebrations . . . when I bow my head and turn away. Tears crash down my cheeks, and all I can do is remember how deeply I love and miss you."

—DR. JOANNE CACCIATORE

Happiness and sadness mix together and seeing so much delight can be a painful thing. It feels odd to be crying when others are laughing. We are lucky when we have people who accept us with both our smiles and our tears.

Day Five

"Whether I'm dreaming or I'm awake, on his birthday or on all other days, my whole life has been contaminated with the fact that he is dead."

—JEAN HEGLAND

With everything I do, my life is contaminated by the fact that my husband is dead. And yet . . . my life is also blessed by our love and the time we shared together. Can the blessing cleanse the contamination? Many moments it does. I have to notice the blessing and hold it tightly in my heart.

Day Six

"The calendar isn't measured by the names of the months or seasons anymore, but by those significant dates. The day we met. The first time we kissed. The first dinner with his family. The anniversary of his death. The date of his funeral."

—KRISTAN HIGGINS

After eight years, I forgot the date of my husband's death. I was filling out a form and wrote down July 13th instead of the actual date, July 17th. I interpreted this as an odd kind of healing. In May, June, and July, I often find myself feeling sad, overwhelmed, or confused. Then I remember. This was my husband's dying time. When we ignore dates, our body reminds us. And yet, the calendar has a way of returning to normal in a parallel time. We have all the significant dates, but we also have the return of simple days and months.

Day Seven

"They wrap [holidays] up all neatly with a turkey and clever gifts and lots of eggnog and laugh and laugh, but at the end of the day there are always people missing from the table. And you have to either sit with those empty chairs and laugh, or you can choose not to come to the table at all. I would rather come to the table."

—JULIE BUXBAUM

Things change over time. Once I preferred staying home alone, now I come to the table. My husband and I got married on my birthday. It was my daughter singing, "Unhappy birthday to you" that made me laugh and opened a door to celebrating a birthday that is also my wedding anniversary. I do make time the next day to be alone in case I need to collapse under the weight of the loneliness. Hopefully our grief work gives us a space to let what we want and need change as we change.

Becoming a Grief Whisperer

Choose a holiday to write about. At the top of the page, write, "How can I honor you today?" What did you do with your loved one on this holiday? Did you maintain traditions that you created together or that were passed down through family? Write about the feelings you have, knowing your loved one will not be present with you.

Now, write one way to celebrate. Will you make up a new tradition? Will you continue a shared tradition, modify it, or completely change it? You might choose to help someone less fortunate on that day. You might make the holiday about someone else (I make Valentine's Day about my granddaughter instead of my husband). You might spend the day reading things they wrote or writing to them or about them. If you can't think of anything you want to do, write a message such as, "I love you. I miss you. You're my heart. Always." Wait as long as you need to, and then try again.

Physical Symptoms

Grief is not illness, but it can cause illness. There is medical proof that the level of stress caused by grieving can cause health issues ranging from emotional reactions like depression or panic attacks to physical problems such as generalized muscle pain, flu-like symptoms, or more serious illnesses. It is at times when self-care seems difficult that it is most important.

Day One

"Loss of someone we love cannot be adequately expressed with words . . . the parts of our brain that process physical pain overlap with the neural centers that record social ruptures and rejection."

—DANIEL J. SIEGEL

The physical and emotional pain we feel when someone we love dies is not imaginary. We must respect our own pain and care for ourselves. For me, at first this meant just staying alive. Then it became finding people who could understand and support me. Each person must find their own way.

Day Two

"No one ever told me how sorrow traumatizes your heart, making you think it will never beat exactly the same way again. No one ever told me how grief feels like a wet sock in my mouth. One I'm forced to breathe through, thinking that with each breath I'll come up short and suffocate."

—SARAH NOFFKE

Some people experience panic attacks and rapid breathing. Breathing can slow. Sometimes people experience an irregular heartbeat. The stress hormones that grief releases can cause actual cardiac problems. There is a growing body of information on the physical as well as psychological effects of the trauma of the great sorrow of grief.

Day Three

"Researchers have discovered that [grief, distress, fear, worry, and anger] cause the release of chemicals from the brain called neuropeptides . . . Once this happens, harmful microbes or cancer cells can invade any tissue in the body."

—DR. CASS INGRAM

Grief releases chemicals that can weaken our immune systems. Without necessarily knowing how this is affecting us, it is important to build up our immune systems so we have the energy it takes to be grief warriors.

Day Four

"Your mother died of a condition known as Takotsubo Cardiomyopathy. This is commonly referred to as 'broken heart syndrome.' She couldn't bear to live without your father . . . I tried the best I could, but I couldn't put it back together again."

—JAMIE SCHOFFMAN

Since broken heart syndrome does exist, I'm not sure why I haven't died from it. Many people believe their heart has been damaged by grief. In some cases, it actually has been. Some people die soon after the person they love died. I have mixed feelings. I want to be with my husband, but I also would have missed so much if I had died in 2009.

Day Five

"We are limited beings. We can only handle so much stress, loss, and tragedy . . . Anxiety and panic attacks are common. Anxiety is a natural expression of our grief."

—GARY ROE

There are medications for anxiety and panic attacks, but meditation and other remedies are also helpful. If seeking professional help, it is important to find someone who does not increase your stress by thinking of grief as an illness. Grief is a normal process. It is only that sometimes this process can cause anxiety or illness. We need understanding, not blame or criticism.

Day Six

"Grief frequently leads to changes in the endocrine, immune, autonomic nervous, and cardiovascular systems; all of these are fundamentally influenced by brain function and neurotransmitters."

—JOAN DIDION

When we say that grief damages us, we are telling a physical as well as an emotional truth. Because all of these systems are influenced by brain function and neurotransmitters, grief work can include finding ways to change what we are feeling by changing what we are thinking.

Day Seven

"If it be a point of humanity for man to bring health and comfort to man, and especially to mitigate and assuage the grief of others . . . why may it not then be said that nature does provoke every man to do the same to himself?"

—THOMAS MORE

We must learn to give ourselves the gentle care we give to others or to our animals. Are there small changes we can make in our day that will increase our wellness? Are their large changes we can make? We could join a gym or train for a marathon. We must take care of our bodies, but also our minds. Taking gentle care of ourselves unexpectedly brings forward the possibility of joy and pleasure as part of our grief journey.

Becoming a Grief Whisperer

If you have continuing physical symptoms, please see a doctor who understands grief. Make a medical wellness checklist. Consider both Western and holistic medicine, things that build physical strength and your immune system, and things that reduce stress. Your list might include yoga, acupuncture, a physical exam, Reiki, swimming, dancing, meditation, hypnosis, and vitamins. The list can include things you have done before and things you might want to try. Now, pick one thing from your list. Do it as an experiment to see if your feeling of wellness increases. Then, try something else. Learn slowly to take care of yourself the way your loved one would take care of you. It can also be helpful to see a grief counselor.

WEEK 39
Signs

Many grievers believe they receive signs from the dead. Others want to receive signs but don't find any. Some believe the idea of signs is imaginary foolishness. Are there things we cannot see because we're not looking in the right place, or things that simply do not exist? On my husband's first birthday after his death, I bought him a cupcake with a candle. His spirit did not blow out the candle as I had hoped. Then I randomly opened a book. Inside the book was an unremembered note from him that said, "I love you. Don't be insecure or I'll cry. I adore you." Coincidence or sign? Coincidence and sign?

Day One

"And after that, when days have gone by, keep an eye out for me. I might write on the steam in the mirror when you're having a bath, or play with the leaves on the apple tree when you're out in the garden. I might slip into a dream."

—JENNY DOWNHAM

Keep an eye out. If you don't believe in signs, you won't see them. If you believe in them but aren't paying attention, you might miss them. What did you notice or fail to notice today that might be a sign from someone you love?

Day Two

"If your husband died, and he loved cardinals, and on the anniversary of his death you happen to walk out to his memorial and you find a cardinal sitting on it, you are allowed to take this as a sign."

—EBEN ALEXANDER

Many believe that cardinals specifically are signs from the dead. Also bluebirds. We had a cardinal that lived near our house that we named Rita (after Rita Hayworth). I sometimes wonder if Rita is at our old house looking for me. All that matters is, we are allowed to interpret anything we want as a sign if it brings us comfort or enriches our lives.

Day Three

"After our loved ones cross over, they are very anxious to let us know they are okay and are aware of what is going on in our lives. If we are not able to feel them around us, they will often give us signs that we cannot ignore . . . They place common objects such as feathers, coins, or rocks in our path . . . that were significant to them."

—KAREN NOE

Feathers, coins, rocks. All signs? I asked a religious figure once if my loved ones still cared for me. He said yes. When I show doubt that something is a sign, many people tell me it definitely is. Our loved ones are persistent. If we are unable to see their messages, they keep trying.

Day Four

"Fragrance may be one of the strongest ways to know that a deceased family member or friend is nearby. People commonly report smelling their perfume or cologne. Some say they still catch whiffs of that person's unique smell . . . "

—PHIL MUTZ

There are certain scents associated with the people we love. Some people have a sense of these scents lingering, far past the time when they could still exist naturally in the air. I tend to hear and feel things rather than experiencing scents. I wonder if what appears to us has to do with the intention of our loved one, or if it is part of our own interpretation.

Day Five

"The percentage of people reporting contact with the dead . . . ranges anywhere from 42 to 72 percent . . . But a sad 75 percent of all those who had encounters reported not mentioning them to anyone for fear of ridicule. It's hard to believe that a society can deny the validity of an experience shared by so large a proportion of its population."

—JULIA ASSANTE

It surprises me how many people report having contact with the dead. Perhaps if we talked about it more, people would feel safe to share their own experiences. I sometimes discount my own experiences with my husband as wishful thinking, but it is more difficult to discount people I have just met who say they see him with me, or friends who never met him who report contact with them. A friend who started meditating said he heard my husband encouraging him.

Day Six

"Whatever the sign is, it will instantly have a connection, or a bridge, to a memory . . . these can be dates, times, locations, or something that brings back an instant memory of an experience that you had with your loved one."

—BLAIR ROBERTSON

There are as many different kinds of signs as there are loved ones. What do you think is something unique to your loved one that they might want you to feel or see or hear or smell that you would know was a sign just from them?

Day Seven

"Grief brings us great pain, but the Other Side teaches us that this pain is not about the absence of love—it's about the continuation of that love. The brilliant cords of love that connect us to someone in this life endure into the afterlife. And when we feel unbearable pain at the loss of a loved one, it is like we are tugging on that cord of love. The pain is real because the cord is real."

—LAURA LYNNE JACKSON

Signs, whether you see them or not, are a symbol of love. We grieve because we continue to love and I believe we continue to be loved. The cord of love stretching between this world and the next is strong. We tug to say, "show me you still love me." They tug to say, "I still love you. I know you are hurting but I am still here." If you think that at the end of life there is only decay and dust, the cord is still there. It is the cord of the love you hold in your own heart that keeps the relationship, if not the person, alive.

Becoming a Grief Whisperer

Close your eyes. Picture yourself somewhere calm and beautiful. You could be walking in a forest or along the beach, or sitting in front of a warming fire. Now, picture signs all around you. If you don't see any, pick something you would like to see and place it wherever you want. If you are in a forest, you might see a fawn or a brightly colored leaf. If you are on a beach, you might see a shiny shell, or a whale in the distance. If you are sitting by a cozy fire, you might notice a book you liked to read together. When you come out of this experience and resume your regular day, look around. When you see different things, merely ask the question, "Is it a sign?" I wonder what answer you will receive.

Honoring Our Dead

We are the rememberers. We are the keepers of their stories.
One of the ways we can create meaning in a life that feels devoid
of meaning is to honor our beloved dead. We can set up grave-
stones and shrines. We can make donations to charity in their
name. We can live double, for them and for ourselves, and see
things with their eyes as well as our own. Many people make
it their life's work to dedicate time and energy to something
important to their beloved dead. I make myself available to other
grieving people; this honors the way my husband made himself
available to addicts and alcoholics.

Day One

"I missed her so much that I wanted to build a
hundred-foot memorial to her with my bare hands . . .
Everybody passing could comprehend how much I
miss her. How physical my missing is."

—MAX PORTER

If you are ever made to feel that you are doing too much to honor your
beloved dead, remember that the Taj Mahal is a tomb. The Egyptian pyr-
amids are tombs. From the beginning of time, people all over the world
have remembered those they love by building monuments to them. Why?
Because our missing is the biggest thing there is, and it lasts forever.

Day Two

"Let's put the fun back in funeral!"

—KRESLEY COLE

Why not? There is sadness at funerals but also the fun of remembering.
I gave away my husband's T-shirts and many of his books at the celebration of his life. I remember looking up and seeing all these people wearing
his shirts and carrying his books. The food was good. The best part was
the stories. Some poignant, but many funny. My husband was an imperfect man loved by many, especially me. I'm for putting the fun back in
funeral and also finding a way to put some fun into the lonely grieving
that comes after.

Day Three

"The funerary banquet celebrates a life . . . and the victory is in overcoming and accepting the change that death brings; honoring a loved one at death becomes victorious because it renews the living."

—JACQUELINE S. THURSBY

I wonder if the funeral is the end or the beginning. I wonder if it is a day to
say goodbye or a day to say hello. Perhaps the way we honor and remember our loved ones at their funeral is the first moment of our learning to
honor them every day for the rest of our lives. It is our victory and our
renewal to live on, to honor, and to love.

Day Four

"The answer to feeling more peaceful is to bring my awareness back to the present moment, to commit to taking actions that honor my intention to live a good life and to make the world a better place, and that by doing so I am honoring my parents and friends who have died, and that as a result, they are still with me."

—CLAIRE BIDWELL SMITH

Can we hold hands with our dead? Can we bring a circle of love into the present moment so that everything we do to make our lives full and make the world a better place is something we do not alone, but with those we love? This is how we keep them alive in our hearts—and in the world.

Day Five

"Across the globe, even in the world's 'worst places,' people found ways to turn pain into wisdom and suffering into strength. They made their own actions, their very lives, into a memorial that honored the people they had lost."

—ERIC GREITENS

There is death everywhere. How can we transform our reactions to this horrible fact so that even in the worst places, in the worst times, we live our lives not in stillness and hiding but in open joy? How can we make our life a memorial to those who have gone before, and make their life matter more than their death?

Day Six

"Because they may be gone, but I'm not. I honor their memories by living, not by becoming the walking dead."

— ANNE CALHOUN

Someone called it "zombie grief." Numb and in pain we can stumble through life, empty and waiting to die. Or, we can honor the lives of those we love by learning how to be fully alive. I do not leave my loved ones behind. I take them with me every step of my way.

Day Seven

"The way I will truly honor my (loved one's) memory is not with a big act, but through my daily choices: to be compassionate with myself . . . to give myself freely to those I love . . . and to live fully and completely while I have the chance."

—CAMILLE PAGÁN

What can I learn from the life my husband lived? If I take his hand, he will guide me forward. I don't have to do big things. If I smile at someone, If I make a small gesture, that may be enough. On my husband's birthday and on the anniversary of his death, I ask people to do acts of kindness to keep his smile going. I want every day to be a day I keep his smile going.

Becoming a Grief Whisperer

On a piece of paper or in your journal, write, "I honor you." Follow that with "I honor you by . . . " and think of something you are doing that honors your loved one. It may be as small as "I honor you by breathing when it hurts to breathe" or as big as, "I honor you by creating a foundation in your name." Then write, "I will honor you by . . . " This is something you would like to do in the future to honor your loved one. It might be, "I will honor you by making a collage of your pictures" or "I will honor you by walking every day." Write as little or as much as you want. You can plant a garden or draw a picture. You can do something alone or with other people. As with all Becoming a Grief Whisperer exercises, however you choose to do this will be exactly the right way.

WEEK 41
Creating Meaning

When someone we love dies, it may seem as though grief drains our lives of all meaning. I believe that I am still alive, whether I want to be or not, because I have work still to do here on Earth. For me, meaning comes from supporting other grievers to honor my husband's work as a recovering alcoholic. Meaning also comes from my relationships to others. This can be friends or family but it can also be my wider community that I try to be of service to. I believe each of us can find meaning if we look into our hearts.

Day One

"He would not want us to walk away from this room weeping and mourning . . . He would want us to walk away celebrating his life, happy for all that he brought to us, and he would want us to be determined. Determined to live our lives the way he lived. With passion and purpose."

—KAREN KINGSBURY

In our sorrow, we may forget that our loved ones can still inspire us. If we are determined to find passion and purpose, it will help us survive our grief. It can be working against bullying after a beloved child's suicide or working to raise cancer awareness after a beloved one's death from cancer. Or simply being more loving to your family or rescuing an animal. What in your loved one's life or death can help you find meaning in your own life?

Day Two

"For now is my grief heavier than the sands of the seas . . . this world has emptied me of all but the oldest purpose: tomorrow's life."

— FRANK HERBERT

From the moment we take our first breath, life has a purpose for us. Until our last breath, we each day find our way to fulfill the oldest purpose. Tomorrow's life is coming. What will we do to make that life mean something to ourselves and others?

Day Three

"Healing is not about moving on or 'getting over it,' it's about learning to make peace with our pain and finding purpose in our lives again."

—SHIRLEY KAMISKY

I don't see healing as an end point but as a process. Moving on or getting over it is, in many cases, impossible and even irrelevant. In making peace with our pain, we are supported by our ability to find purposeful meaning once again. The person we love may have died, but the meaning our love gives us has not.

Day Four

"Every muscle aches; my heart most of all . . . It hurts worse than anything. I don't know how I'm supposed to be expected to live carrying this kind of pain . . . I want to stop running away from everything. I want to find something to run toward."

—HANNAH HARRINGTON

Grief and missing can blast our lives to pieces. We don't know how to live when we carry such a weight of pain. This can make us want to run away from everything. It is our responsibility to begin to find things to run toward. Often we do this by feeling our loved ones pull us back into life.

Day Five

"It is said that life . . . is like a mosaic made of countless tiny stones. Each person's life comprises a part of the mosaic, and each person can only see their part of the mosaic . . . All the pain, sweat, and grief that are the lot of every man—those are the stones man is given power to place."

—CHRISTOPHER BUNN

My stones are broken pieces. They have rough edges. They are the result of much that has been shattered. Still, their shapes and colors call to me. How can I put them together again, not to create the old picture, but to create a new mosaic that represents the grief and pain, and also the beauty and love?

Day Six

"This is what those who haven't crossed the tropic of grief often fail to understand: the fact that someone is dead may mean that they are not alive, but doesn't mean that they do not exist."

—JULIAN BARNES

We may find that at the same time our loved one's death creates a sense of meaninglessness, their continued existence in our hearts, minds, and souls creates a way for us to redefine meaning in our life. It's a bit of a puzzle. I feel my husband is both absent and present. It is a daily renewal of my commitment to him and to his love of life to keep trying to find meaning and then to take actions that will have a meaningful impact on both my life and the lives of others.

Day Seven

"When those you love die, the best you can do is honor their spirit for as long as you live . . . take whatever lesson that person or animal was trying to teach you, and you make it true in your own life . . . keep their spirit alive in the world, by keeping it alive in yourself."

—PATRICK SWAYZE

That's the secret of the gift. What are the lessons that I am meant to learn? What was I given by sharing this deep love? How can I best honor my husband's spirit by keeping him alive in my heart but also by keeping his spirit and his work alive in the world?

Becoming a Grief Whisperer

Once a day, for as many days as you find helpful, write "I am still alive. My life has meaning." Write it 10 or more times. If you are comfortable with this, write on a mirror you look into often. "I am still alive. My life has meaning."

At any point in the day or night when you have thoughts about what that meaning might be, notice them and write them down. Ask your loved one what part of their life they would like you to keep alive in the world for them. Imagine what they would say. It might take a second, it might take longer, but you will start feeling a sense of meaning returning. As you do, you will also discover what actions you need to take to give this meaning life.

Showing Up

When consumed by grief, it's natural to isolate and lack motivation to participate in the world. It is much more comfortable to stay at home with our sorrow and memories. I began to show up for things, whether I wanted to or not, hoping that life would seep back into me. Sometimes nothing much happened. I went out, suffered through the event, and was glad to go home again. In spite of myself, in time I found myself smiling. In time, I found myself meeting a new person I found interesting. I allowed myself to come alive again. Even now, I sometimes have to force myself to show up. I am working on looking forward to things. My grief can come with me wherever I go.

Day One

"I'm just a butterfly, a mourning cloak, sealed inside a cocoon with blind eyes and sticky wings. And suddenly I wonder if the cocoons sometimes do not open, if the butterfly inside is ever simply not strong enough to break through."

—ALLY CONDIE

Grief can undermine our belief in our own possibility. It weakens us. To live in such a way that, instead of trying to reach our full potential, we imprison ourselves in our private cocoon of grief, is a sad denial of our very nature. How can we find that will to break through, stretch our wings, and fly? I think we do it with remembered love.

Day Two

"Not only are there many ways to grieve, but showing sorrow, reaching out, being honest about your loss is as important as anything . . . Go celebrate your own life before it's over."

—KRIS RADISH

I want to learn to celebrate my own life because you love me. If you love me, there must be something still inside me worth celebrating. I can get to the joy by being authentic about the sorrow. I show up with the fullness of my being even while I grieve.

Day Three

"I was scared of living a life not worth the living. Why did I deserve to live when my sister had died? I was responsible now for two lives, my sister's and my own, and, damn, I'd better live well."

—NINA SANKOVITCH

From the very moment that my husband took his last breath I have felt this responsibility. I live now not only for myself, but for him. I want to take everything he has given me and figure out how to love life as he did, and live life for both of us with as many breaths as I have left.

Day Four

"Outside has everything. Whenever I think of a thing now like skis or fireworks or islands or elevators or yo-yos, I have to remember they're real, they're actually happening in Outside all together. It makes my head tired. And people too, firefighters teachers burglars babies saints soccer players and all sorts, they're all really in Outside. I'm not there, though."

—EMMA DONOGHUE

"Outside" can be a scary place. There is so much "Outside" to show up for. It is okay to sometimes not be ready. There are a lot of things inside as well. You will show up for "Outside" when you are ready. You may already be ready but just not notice it yet. That happens. Sometimes the first step seems so difficult, it is better to start with the seventh step because then you are already on your way.

Day Five

"What he feared the most was that all this hiding had made it impossible for him to ever be found again."

—JOHN COREY WHALEY

When hiding becomes all that you know, the fear of coming into view again can be overwhelming. What is lost can be found, but it does not always feel that way. That's why showing up can begin by simply going for a two-minute walk. Remember when you come out of your hiding place you can always go back in. Respect your fear, and then follow it to see where it leads you.

Day Six

"Feel. Grieve. Just sit and let it all rip you apart. And then get up and keep breathing. One breath at a time. One day at a time. Wake up, and be shredded. Cry for a while. Then stop crying and go about your day. You're not okay but you're alive."

—JASINDA WILDER

You don't have to wait to be okay to show up. You don't have to let go to find a thing or two to do. If you accidentally find yourself having a happy moment, there will be time to cry later. It is not disloyal to live while you are alive. Part of showing up is learning how to dance again, even if it is with a certain silly awkwardness.

Day Seven

"We can remain gray and immobile in the wake of our losses or we can open ourselves up to the world, let the sunshine in, fill our surroundings with heaps of flowers, and know that we loved someone truly and deeply."

—CLAIRE BIDWELL SMITH

Showing up is a way of saluting the love we have. What a gift, to love someone truly and deeply. Do we say thank you for that gift by retreating from the world? We can. Or we can say thank you for that gift by opening our windows and letting in the fresh air of life. You can't bring me flowers any more, but I can bring myself flowers. It's not the same life, but your love can continue to make it a blessed life, if I show up for it.

Becoming a Grief Whisperer

Make three lists. List 10 things you used to like to do but haven't done since the one you love died. List 10 things you would like to do but have never done. List 10 things that intrigue you but you think you wouldn't try. If you can't write 10 things, you can write 7 or 3 or 14. Pick one thing from any of the three lists and put it on your calendar. You may find yourself doing it, or not. Each week, pick one or more things to put on your calendar. In time, you might find that you are not only enjoying something that you forced yourself to do, you are looking forward to it.

Helping Others

When I do something to help another human being or animal I turn my attention to them. Helping others is essential to my grief journey. When I was very withdrawn I could use the Internet to write encouraging posts to people. Some of these people became friends. It was something that took very little energy and was beneficial to them but also to me.

Day One

"I'm not really here to keep you from freaking out. I'm here to be with you while you freak out, or grieve or laugh or suffer or sing. It is a ministry of presence. It is showing up with a loving heart."

—KATE BRAESTRUP

Helping others may seem overwhelming if we think we need to be a problem solver when what is really needed is the presence of a loving heart. That presence creates the connection and support, and, in time, change

Day Two

"I couldn't do anything at all except feed her, hold her when she cried, pray angry prayers, keep showing up, and hope that time and my home and presence would offer healing."

—GLENNON DOYLE MELTON

Grief begs to be heard. To have someone care without denying the validity of your grief is a blessing. To help someone means to show up. Showing up is not always easy when you are grieving yourself, but shared grief has much solace in it.

Day Three

"I show my scars so that others know they can heal."

—RHACHELLE NICOL'

It is natural to want to keep our scars hidden. I never thought I would show mine so openly. In making a space to share scars we are all helped to find our way through grief.

Day Four

"Holding the space doesn't mean swaddling the family immobile in their grief. It also means giving them meaningful tasks . . . Activities give the mourner a sense of purpose. A sense of purpose helps the mourner grieve. Grieving helps the mourner begin to heal."

—CAITLIN DOUGHTY

When someone we love dies, our lives can feel meaningless. Helping others starts to give us back our sense of purpose. This can be simple, like cooking a meal or taking a walk with someone who is mourning. It can be more complicated, like helping a griever choose which belongings to keep and which to pack up and give away. As we do things together, our grief doesn't go away, but the shape of it begins to change.

Day Five

"Those who can sit in silence with their fellow man . . . can bring new life in a dying heart. Those who are not afraid to hold a hand in gratitude, to shed tears in grief, and to let a sigh of distress arise straight from the heart, can break through paralyzing boundaries and witness the birth of a new fellowship, the fellowship of the broken."

—HENRI J.M. NOUWEN

We can be a passive member of the "fellowship of the broken," or we can be an active member. No one wants to join this group, but we were not given a choice. Sitting with others creates a bond with the living as well as with the dead. You don't need to know what to say. Listening is enough.

Day Six

"It's so dark right now; I can't see any light around me. That's because the light is coming from you. You can't see it but everyone else can."

—LANG LEAV

Grief makes everything dark. However, there is still a light coming from you. It is the light of your struggling life force and the light of your love. Part of grief work is finding that light and learning where to shine it. By giving it to others, you receive it yourself.

Day Seven

"When we share in each other's grief and pain, we lighten it . . . Like the rain, tears too have an end. And with deep emotions, we are open to each other in unexpected ways."

—KARPOV KINRADE

There are many grievers. We can find them in person, in groups, or just in the world. We can find them online. Helping others by sharing our own grief makes a connection. We begin to see that we are not crazy and we are not alone. There is comfort in acceptance. There is unexpected growth of seedlings of life if we take the risk of opening ourselves up.

Becoming a Grief Whisperer

Think about what kind of help you might like to give. You may want to stay in the virtual world, but it is also good to venture out into the real world. You may want to work with other grievers, or with animals. You may want to tend a community garden or deliver meals to elderly people. If your first idea doesn't work, try your second and third ideas. You can be the person that makes a difference in another's life. That will make a difference in your life.

It Happens Every Day

One of the reasons people tell you to "get over it" or "move on" is that they think grief is fixed in time. They know the person you love died a year ago or five years ago or even 40 years ago, and they think you are stuck. They don't understand that the trauma of grief happens over and over every day as we live with the constant reminder that the person we love so much will never be here again to share our lives. We can learn to live with this trauma in healthy and happy ways, but we can't stop the feelings from assailing us in new and yet familiar ways.

Day One

"Every time I take a breath or blink or speak, I experience her death all over again. I don't sit here and wonder if the fact that she's dead will ever sink in. I sit here and wonder when I'll stop having to watch her die."

—COLLEEN HOOVER

Some of us actually see and feel the moment of our loved one's death over and over again. That doesn't happen to me, but I remember every detail of my husband's dying time. Even after eight years I have so many moments where I have to remind myself that my husband is dead. I know he's dead, but I still experience it in fresh ways. Everyone dies. I know that. It still doesn't make sense.

Day Two

"Here is one of the worst things about having someone you love die: It happens again every single morning."

—ANNA QUINDLEN

When we wake up, often our first thought is that our beloved is no longer alive. We have to get through another day without them. Instead of getting up easily and with joy, we have to find a way to remember their death and yet be so inspired by their life that we find the energy to start our day. Some days this is easy; other days it seems impossible.

Day Three

"But as the years passed, he missed her more, not less, and his need for her became a cut that would not scar over, would not stop leaking."

—DENNIS LEHANE

People who have not suffered deep grief often think that missing someone is something we get used to. Grief is exhausting because many of us miss our loved ones more with each passing day. We need to keep changing the bandage on our wound. We need to live with it because we find it incurable.

Day Four

"I decide this is just A Bad Day. We all get them, because grief doesn't care how many years it's been."

—SARA BARNARD

I will say today is "A Bad Day." I sleep too much or watch too much television. Even the simplest things seem impossible. Sometimes a bad day can turn into a good day if I make myself take action. Other times it just has to be accepted as a bad day, with the hope that tomorrow will be a better one.

Day Five

"You start to understand that grief is chronic. That it's more about remission and relapse than it is about a cure . . . you can't simply wait for it to be over. You have to move through it, like swimming in an undertow."

—TAYLOR JENKINS REID

While I know people who feel they have been released from grief, for me it is chronic. My grief won't end until I take my last breath. I have moments when I feel alive and strong, and moments when I collapse under the weight of it. What I have learned over the years is not to succumb to it, but rather to call it out and keep moving as much as I can. I have to be a better swimmer.

Day Six

"It's funny how, even long after you've accepted the grief of losing someone you love and truly have gotten on with your life . . . something comes up that plays 'gotcha,' and for a moment or two the scar tissue separates and the wound is raw again."

—MARY HIGGINS CLARK

Grief can surprise us with its renewed intensity. It is not taking a step backward when the scar tissue separates and the wound is raw again, even if the feeling lasts an hour, a day, or a week. Grief ebbs and flows. It may gentle down but it rarely disappears completely.

Day Seven

"Grief doesn't sink into the shadows the moment the sun comes up. You can't sleep your way through misery. There are some hurts that become a part of you, like your blood or your eyes or your teeth . . . "

—AUTUMN DOUGHTON

Grief is in my bones. It is part of who I am. Some days I make it my companion, and some days I am again wounded by it. My work has been to find a home for it so I can live a magical and wonderful life at the same time.

Becoming a Grief Whisperer

Write about or illustrate your grief as you would like it to be, not how it actually is. If you had a magic wand, what would your grief feel like moment by moment? Write a letter to your grief. Start with, "Dear Grief." Do you want your grief to vanish completely? Are there lessons your grief teaches you? Do you want to ask it questions, or express your anger and impatience with it? Do you want it to stay but only as a reminder of love and happiness, without the attached fear and pain? Tell your grief what you wish from it, and ask your grief to grant those wishes. You can sign the letter "With Love" followed by your name, or not.

Was It Worth It?

Over the years, only one person I have asked has said no. I have learned to be grateful for my grief. The depth of my grief measures the height of my love. I would not give up one moment with my husband. The time we had together is more than worth the suffering I have experienced since his death.

Day One

"The more loss we feel, the more grateful we should be for whatever it was we had to lose. It means that we had something worth grieving for. The ones I'm sorry for are the ones that go through life not knowing what grief is."

—FRANK O'CONNOR

How lucky I am to love and be loved. I am blessed that I was given something to lose. I do feel sorry for people who never have this love and therefore never know grief. While I grieve deeply for my husband, I had a difficult relationship with my parents and was relieved when they died. I find that lack of grief much sadder than grief itself.

Day Two

"No one cries very much unless something of real worth is lost. So grieving is a celebration of the depth of the union. Tears are the jewels of remembrance— sad but glistening with the beauty of the past."

—SUSAN J. ZONNEBELT-SMEENGE

If we remember the deep worth of the relationship we have had and the beautiful moments it contained, the next step is to make our celebration of that more important than the deprivation we feel now. Consider the words, "Grieving is a celebration." What does that sentence mean to you? What can it begin to mean?

Day Three

"Although it seemed impossible to find joy in the depths of her grief . . . this hurt she felt was the price of loving with her whole heart. But having Gran in her life had been worth every moment of pain."

—SUSAN WIGGS

To have people in our lives whom we love with our whole heart is something not everyone has. To think of it as a blessing, even after they have died, is a solace. My moments of joy and deep understanding with my husband are worth every moment of the pain I feel now.

Day Four

"I try to remember the woman she was and not the
woman I have built out of spare parts to comfort me
in my mourning. And . . . as the days go by and the
balm of my forgiveness washes over the cracked and
parched surface of my heart, I find that remembering
her as she was is a gift I can give us both."

—CAROLYN PARKHURST

Someone told me soon after my husband died that in a while, I would only
have good memories. I replied that I wanted to remember him as he really
was, not in an idealized way. In his dying time, my husband apologized for
all the ways he had failed me. I apologized too. I still get angry with him. I
still wish we both had been better at expressing our love. Forgiveness still
comes. True and honest remembrance of how we tried and how we suc-
ceeded, how we tried and how we failed, is a gift. All of it was worth it.
Every moment was worth it.

Day Five

"Would I forgo the pleasure of her company to escape
the bleakness of her loss . . . Not for a moment . . .
I shall be richer all my life for this sorrow."

—WALLACE STEGNER

Though I would prefer not to have it at all, my sorrow makes my life
richer. The pleasure of this deeply connected and loving relationship
far outweighs the pain of grief.

Day Six

"I am too full of the sun to be mournful of the rain."

—VINATI BHOLA

I am full of the sun of your love. I am still mournful of the rain. Maybe someday I will be able to dance in the rain.

Day Seven

"Grief is existential testimony to the worth of the one loved. That worth abides. So I own my grief. I do not try to put it behind me, to get over it, to forget it . . . Every lament is a love-song."

—NICHOLAS WOLTERSTORFF

Every tear, every curse, is a testament to how special you are, to how much you will always be worth to me. I am proud to be a griever. I do not want to be healed. I want to live always full of the knowledge of you and what our life together meant and continues to mean to me and to others.

Becoming a Grief Whisperer

Write or record a story of your loved one who has died. Tell the tale of experiences you shared, of things they did in the world. Make them come alive again through your words. You can laugh or cry while you do this. You can laugh and cry at the same time. When you have finished, rest for a while. Then ask yourself: Is knowing this person and loving them worth the grief you are experiencing now? If the answer is yes, don't be afraid to continue to tell their story, to others or just to yourself.

Standing Up for Grief

It is acceptable to be silent about grief in order to avoid hurtful comments from others. However, what if you tried to educate people by standing up for your grief? Let them know that grief, with all its twists and turns, is a normal response to death. Grief is not complicated or prolonged. It just is. It is time we started acknowledging grief rather than denying it. If you are more comfortable in silence, be reassured that it's okay to stand up for your own grief in private moments. You have the right to grieve in your own time, in your own way.

Day One

"As a culture, we seem to have an intolerance for suffering . . . by minimizing the impact of significant losses, pathologizing those whose reactions are intense, and applauding those who seem relatively unaffected by tragic events, we encourage the inhibition of our own grief."

—H. NORMAN WRIGHT

I embrace authenticity of emotion. I do not consider stoicism a virtue. When my husband was dying, I was as glad he could cry with me as I was that he could laugh with me. Grief is not something to be stuffed down or hidden. It is especially dangerous when people want to pathologize grief. I applaud those who have the courage to remove their mask and those who are willing to honor and share the genuine process and expression of grief.

Day Two

"The natural response . . . because it is uncomfortable to them to hear the grieving person crying, is to try to get the person to stop crying and cheer them up. That is really the wrong approach . . . it is important that the person be allowed to grieve so the healing process can begin."

—KEVIN M. GARDNER

I learned in a workshop that when someone was crying, not to offer them a tissue or try to comfort them, but rather to sit quietly and witness their tears. Unhappiness often makes other people uncomfortable, and they react by trying to cheer up the person suffering. Instead of bringing cheer, their comments cause hurt, irritation, and confusion. Grief is an honorable emotion reflecting love, and before healing can start, it must be heard and respected.

Day Three

"Today, in our 'shut up, get over it, and move on' mentality, our society misses so much, it's no wonder we are a generation that longs to tell our stories."

—ELISABETH KÜBLER-ROSS

When we are forbidden by societal norms from telling our honest story, we miss so much. Instead of walking through life arm in arm with shared emotional experience, we feel isolated and alienated. We can shut up or we can speak up. Which choice will make us feel truly alive?

Day Four

"Rather than running from grief's harsh reality, you may find that in letting it groan and pierce and ache and cry, you begin to exhaust some of its staying power. You expose its secret hiding places. You force it into the open air where it can be more easily outlined and dealt with."

—FRANK PAGE

I find groaning, crying, tantrums, and an occasional wallow in grief helpful, but I try to keep this within the privacy of my own home. If I can let out my grief in whatever way I want, it feels cleansing. I have released energy to do other things. I can't deal with what I hide even from myself.

Day Five

"When you lost a family member back then you were supposed to be in full mourning, dress in nothing but black . . . Then you went into something they called 'half mourning' for another full year . . . Now? A month after a tragedy, maybe two, and you're expected to be all better, or down pills so you can pretend you are."

—MERCEDES LACKEY

In most modern cultures, there is no longer an acceptable outward expression of mourning. There is no way for someone to look at us and know how deep our grief is. It may seem that our only choice is to smooth over the cracks in our sense of self by false remedies or even harmful medication. I want to change this expectation. I want everyone to understand that a grieving person is supposed to grieve.

Day Six

"When asked, 'Why do you always wear black?' he said, 'I'm in mourning for my life.'"

—ANTON CHEKHOV

We may not wear black openly, but many of us carry our hearts, minds, and souls draped in black. We are in mourning for a life that continues on after those we love have died. We are mourning for the life we wanted that is no longer possible. We learn to understand that we can be in mourning for our life at the same time we learn to celebrate it. We don't have to let go to move on.

Day Seven

"Just walk fearlessly into the house of mourning, for grief is just love squaring up to its oldest enemy. And after all these mortal human years, love is up to the challenge."

—CATHERINE BURNS

Where do we find the courage to grieve, especially openly? In love. Love moves us from thinking of grief as a curse to considering the idea that grief can be a blessing. As sad and broken as we are, I do believe that love is up to the challenge. In the middle of the worst horror, love can find a way through, if we let it.

Becoming a Grief Whisperer

Using your own experience, write a newspaper or magazine article about grief. It could have a serious tone for an academic journal, or be a chatty piece for the lifestyle section, helpful for others, or even humorous. If you prefer, make a personal film about grief. What do you want people to know? What are your true feelings? How do you want others to respond? What do you never want to hear again? Be as creative as you like. When you finish, you can keep your work for yourself or decide if you want to share it with others.

Finding Solutions

Is grief a problem we should expect to solve? What would a solution look like? We might find that grieving is in itself a solution. Or that there are certain practical things we can do to feel better. You have the right to define "solution" however you wish and not have someone else's definition imposed upon you.

Day One

"If someone describes a griever to me by saying, 'Oh, she's so strong and together; she's handling her grief really well,' that's when I worry. I think someone is handling her grief well if I hear that 'she's terribly upset, she's crying constantly, she's falling apart.' Emotion isn't the problem . . . it's the natural response and the ultimate solution."

— ASHLEY DAVIS BUSH

I find it difficult to talk with someone who is radiating pain and saying they are okay. I find it easy to sit with someone who is honest about how they feel. One cannot begin to treat a wound if they are busy pretending it doesn't exist.

Day Two

"High-tide grief calls for empathy, not solutions."

—DEE BRESTIN

People need to find their own way through grief. It is empathy that opens our hearts, not being told what to do. One solution that inspires the beginnings of healing is being listened to and understood. No one understands exactly how I feel. No one has authority over my experience. Finding people who support me as I look for healthier ways to grieve lightens my burden.

Day Three

"Later, we do an exercise where we write down Trigger Situations and Solutions for how to deal with them. My triggers: morning, evening, happy, sad, nothing, something."

—JOWITA BYDLOWSKA

As experienced as we become with grief, it can still be difficult to know what our triggers are. Sometimes it seems everything is a trigger. However, we can change how we react to a specific trigger. In the beginning, if I saw a sport that my husband loved to watch, I would be angry and sad that it continued without him being alive to enjoy it. Then it occurred to me that I could think instead about how much joy these things had given him while he was alive. You can change the way you feel about things, even grief, by changing what you say to yourself about them.

Day Four

"Sometimes, laughing like a lunatic can be the best solution. Or crying loudly into a pillow. But don't regret anything. Always tell yourself 'I. Regret. Nothing.'"

—VICTORIA ESTRADA

Regret is one of grief's weapons. So many things we could have done better. So many things stolen from our future. But if we say we regret nothing, perhaps we will, in time, lose the sting of regret. Laughter is always a solution for me, as is crying. They express both ends of my emotional range. I search out things that cause me to laugh, but I also search out things that cause me to cry. I find both cleansing.

Day Five

"If art can help us grieve, can help us mourn, then lean on it."

—LIN-MANUEL MIRANDA

To get lost in a painting, a photograph, or any kind of art, is a way of transcending grief. Whatever can become a cushion for my grief to rest on, let me seek it out. Let me remember to lean on it.

Day Six

"To cry in the memory of someone is not a problem at all rather it is a solution."

— NITIN YADUVANSHI

Sometimes what we are defining as problems are really solutions. If I cry in memory of someone, if I spend some time in bed, if I am not over it, perhaps none of these are problems unless I say they are. Maybe they are solutions to help me through another day.

Day Seven

"Disassemble the cells of a sponge . . . then dump them into a solution, and they will find their way back together and build themselves into a sponge again . . . because, like you and me and every other living thing, they have one overwhelming impulse: to continue to be."

— BILL BRYSON

No matter how broken into pieces you feel, there is the possibility of reassembling yourself. Some call it the new normal; others call it the new abnormal. You may feel that with someone else's death, you died too. Yet you continue to be. This is your life force pulsing underneath the cover of your grief. What strategy is required for the reassembling of your own self?

Becoming a Grief Whisperer

Using building blocks, make any kind of structure. Knock it down. Build it again. Knock it down. Build something else. Repeat as many times as you like. Now, just look at the blocks. Think about what you need for building blocks to make a new structure out of what is left of yourself and your life. Draw pictures of blocks (perhaps imperfect squares) and label them with the different skills, activities, feelings you need to build yourself up (perhaps motivation, love, or purpose). When you are knocked down you know what you need to build yourself up again. Is it possible there is something freeing in falling apart or a challenge in forming yourself in a new way?

Come Back

It is the cry of every grieving person: "Come back. I know you can't, but please come back." It is the unendurable thing we must endure, knowing that the one we love so deeply is gone forever. Is there a chance that our loved ones are still with us? If they are, does it matter if they are not with us in the earthly form we delighted in?

Day One

"There was a point when I wanted to say to them, Alright, you have died, I know that, and you've been dead for a while, we have all absorbed this . . . but now it's time for you to come back. You have been away long enough."

—LYDIA DAVIS

We know that our dead cannot come back, yet we long for them to do so. In my family we say, "Our dead haven't come back once to visit. How rude!" We laugh, but underneath there is the undeniable inability to accept on every level that our loved one is never coming home.

Day Two

"When someone is in your heart, they're never truly gone. They can come back to you, even at unlikely times."

—MITCH ALBOM

Our loved ones are never again with us, and they are always with us. We carry our loved ones with us in our hearts.

Day Three

"If the dead can . . . move unseen around those they loved, I shall always be near you . . . and if there be a soft breeze upon your cheek, it shall be my breath; or if the cool air fans your throbbing temple, it shall be my spirit passing by."

—PAUL HOFFMAN

Some people are made uncomfortable by the idea of our loved ones remaining close to us, believing that this does not let them go free to the next realm of existence. Some people believe that there is no consciousness after death. I believe my husband is always near me, and that time and space are different where he is. This allows him to do whatever he needs to do while he is with me and with others who love him. I don't have to understand it or even need it to be true. Believing it gives me a framework of sanity to cope with grief.

Day Four

"What kind of wife would I be if I left your father simply because he was dead?"

—JESS WALTER

I have a lot of dead friends. I am married to a dead man. I wish they were alive. I do believe our relationship continues. I don't believe love and connection end with death. I respect people who choose to let go. I choose to hold on and live fully among the living and the dead.

Day Five

"And then sometimes a day would come . . . when she missed him so fiercely she felt empty, not a woman at all anymore but just a dead tree filled with cold November blow. She felt like that now, felt like hollering his name and hollering him home."

—STEPHEN KING

If only that kind of holler existed. I wish there was a way to holler our dead home, but the earth is no longer their home. There is an emptiness that, however we try to fill it, can only be filled by the homecoming that can never be.

Day Six

"There's a jangle to the music of the dead. I mean that certain something that's so happy and so sad at the same time."

—DANIEL JOSÉ OLDER

I wonder if the dead still make music? I can hear the music of their being. I am happy to remember, and sad that we can no longer make music together in the way of the living.

Day Seven

"My mind, I think, has started to become . . . the room of love for the absent are present, the dead are alive, time is eternal . . . The room of love is the love that holds us all, and it is not ours. It goes back before we were born. It goes all the way back."

—WENDELL BERRY

It has been said that we were connected before we met. There are people in our lives who seem to journey with us throughout eternity. If time is eternal, if love is eternal, then there is a level of being in which no one ever leaves. Death may change someone's form, their outer covering, but they do not leave.

Becoming a Grief Whisperer

Pretend you are in an echo chamber. Yell, "Come back" and hear your cry echo. Write about what it would be like if your loved ones came back. How would it change your life? Now, write about your life going on without your loved ones.

Read the first story looking for clues about the things you can put back into your life to give it some of the pleasure and meaning from the love that you still share. Are there actions you can take on your own that are inspired by the life you had together? Write a new story about how your life will go on as you become more fully alive with grief.

If you believe that your loved ones are still with you, end this exercise by feeling them holding you and accepting you exactly as you are. Thank them for all they give you, even after death. If you believe that your loved ones are not with you in any way, end this exercise by sending them your love and thanking them for all they have given you.

WEEK 49
Resources

There are many resources to help grieving people. These include external resources like counseling, groups, and grief support pages. There are also internal resources—qualities within yourself that you can use for emotional and physical support.

Day One

"If I want to live my ability to be fully present and compassionate, my ability to be with it all—the joy and the sorrow—I must find the ways, the people, the places, the practices that support me in being all I truly am . . . that let me feel the warmth of encouragement against my heart when it is weary."

—ORIAH MOUNTAIN DREAMER

Grief can be a time of discovery. Who are the people, what are the places, ways, and practices that will support us during this time? What do we hold within ourselves that can give us encouragement and support when our hearts are too weary to care? I have to train myself to be present even during the times I most want to hide or run away.

Day Two

"I called a cab, still in my towel. I jumped in the cab before it had even stopped at the gate. I actually said, 'The nearest library with a cutting-edge professional grief- and trauma-therapy section, and step on it.'"

—DAVID FOSTER WALLACE

The library and the bookstore are treasure troves of resources that can be of help to us. Even the search itself is an essential part of beginning to take an active role in caring for ourselves.

Day Three

"When life gets hard, ask Google. Google knows everything."

—EMMA HART

I am old enough to remember when the search for information was difficult and resources were limited. Search engines bring the entire world into our homes. There are hundreds of resources for grievers on the Internet. There are things you can read, groups you can join, and people you can call or e-mail. You can be in contact with people all over the world. There are even bereavement cruises, conferences, and camp programs.

Day Four

"Grief excuses you from dusting, another reason why old ladies mourn for so long when their man dies."

—DI DRINKWATER

Grief can disable you in uncomfortable ways. But, if you have a sense of humor, grief can also get you out of tasks you never did like. One of the most important antidotes to grief is laughter.

Day Five

"Reaching out for help also connects you to other people and strengthens the bonds of love that make life seem worth living again."

—DR. ALAN WOLFELT

What a gift it is to reach out and find people who want to listen and understand how we feel. On my Facebook page (Grief Speaks Out), an American mother whose daughter had been murdered once posted, "I'm international now. I have a friend in Australia and another in Liberia." Whether we find our new friends in our daily lives or online, they can become true grief companions. Grief is a common language across all cultures and belief systems.

Day Six

"I dance. A lot. I work grief and sadness out of my body when I dance, and I bring in joy and rhythm."

—INGA MUSCIO

Dance it out. Sing it out. Play it out. There are so many things we are capable of doing with movement, creativity, and sport that may have been part of our daily lives before grief, or that now have a chance to enter our lives because of grief.

Day Seven

"Confronting our feelings and giving them appropriate expression always takes strength, not weakness . . . It takes strength to face our sadness and to grieve and to let our grief and our anger flow in tears . . . to talk about our feelings and to reach out for help and comfort when we need it."

—FRED ROGERS

Finding resources in the world and in us takes strength and determination. It is not weak to feel and express our feelings. It is not weak to ask for help. It is strength of personality requiring love of self and dignity. If I refuse to give up, I will eventually find what works for me.

Becoming a Grief Whisperer

Go Internet exploring. Put in useful combinations of words, or silly or unusual combinations. When I did this exercise, I put in "Grief Dancing," and found a dance performed by a group of people that was choreographed by a man who experienced the death of multiple people he loved. It was beautiful to watch and made me think of trying expressive dancing myself. Search for things related to grief or anything that might interest you.

Now close your eyes and go exploring for your inner resources. Look at yourself with the eyes of those who love you, as well as your own eyes. Focus on your strengths and allow your weaknesses to float away for a while.

Keep a list of all the resources you think might be helpful, interesting, or fun. When you are ready, you can turn thinking about doing things to support you in your grief into actually doing them. One a week? One a day? Open yourself up even a little and see what flows in.

Hooray for Me

Grief makes you vulnerable, but it is time to notice what you are doing and applaud yourself for it. A Hooray for Me can be as simple as getting out of bed in the morning or taking your dog for a walk. A Hooray for Me can be as complex as hosting a dinner party or going back to work. If you have gotten through another day without the person you love with you, you have accomplished something. Notice what you are doing, not what you aren't doing. Become your own cheerleader. You deserve it.

Day One

"I no longer agree to treat myself with disrespect. Every time a self-critical thought comes to mind, I will forgive the Judge and follow this comment with words of praise, self-acceptance, and love."

—DON RUIZ

I am much too gifted at judging myself. I think of what I didn't do instead of what I did accomplish. My friends would describe me in a totally different way than I describe myself. I wouldn't let anyone else be such a harsh judge of me or of themselves. It is time to respect myself and know that I am doing the best I can. I will forgive my judge and act more loving toward myself.

Day Two

"Self-affirm—build yourself up with honest and genuine praise."

—LORII MYERS

I praise other people. I even give compliments to strangers to help them feel better about their day. We can start giving ourselves the praise we give our friends, our children, our pets. I am living my life one day at a time without my husband. I have been doing this for over eight years. That is a huge accomplishment for me. What is there about you that is worthy of honest and genuine praise?

Day Three

"My intellect was useless; my emotions were dead . . . but from time to time, deep in the thickets of my inner wilderness, I could sense the presence of something that knew how to stay alive even when the rest of me wanted to die. That something was my tough and tenacious soul."

—PARKER J. PALMER

Sometimes in the darkness of grief we feel so totally lost that giving ourselves love and praise seems impossible. However, we each have a tough and tenacious part of us that is clinging on that is worthy of praise. Looking for ways to say Hooray For Me is a way of nurturing the part of us that wants to live fully.

Day Four

> "There is no magic cure, no making it all go away forever. There are only small steps upward; an easier day, an unexpected laugh."

—LAURIE HALSE ANDERSON

Each small step contributes to arriving at a new place. There isn't a magic cure, but there are ways of making life more fulfilling. We can even find laughter again. If we accidentally laugh today, what a wonderful Hooray for Me that is. I like to think that when I laugh, my husband smiles with me. I miss his smile. He wouldn't want me to lose mine as well.

Day Five

> "Nothing is better for self-esteem than survival."

—MARTHA GELLHORN

Survival. That is what every griever is learning. Lying in bed and not moving is survival. Increasing the number of happy and productive moments we have is survival. Making it through another day is a Hooray for Me. My grief work has been to make my survival less of a struggle and more of an adventure. I am traveling alone in uncharted territory. Where will I go and what will I discover when I get there?

Day Six

"Even though I still felt a constant ache, I seemed unknowingly to have traveled a little distance away from that first unbearable pain. I sat up straighter and drew a deep breath, and it was then that I began to believe that I really might make my way through this."

—ANNE TYLER

In the first few months after my husband died, when I was researching suicide, I knew I could not continue to live without him. The pain was too huge, and it was paralyzing me. However, I also could not give the grief to others that had been given to me. I could not take my own life. What was I to do? Just one small thing at a time. After eight years, those small things have added up to a lot I can be proud of. Together we are making our way through this. It looks and feel different for each person, but however alone we feel, we're still striving together. Hooray for Us!

Day Seven

"I have come to accept the real me. I have come to love the real me. I now celebrate the real me."

CHARICE PEMPENGCO

This is not an easy one for most of us. It is a goal to love and celebrate "me" as I am. I am far from perfect, yet I am worthy of love and praise. My husband loved me completely and unconditionally. Is it possible to love myself as he loves me?

Becoming a Grief Whisperer

Use gold stars, stickers, or a stamp with an affirmation that makes you smile. On a calendar or journal, at the end of every day write down a Hooray for Me. Use the words. "Hooray for Me! Today I..." Write as many as you want per day. For each one, give yourself a sticker or stamp. Remember, a Hooray for Me can be as simple as, "Hooray For Me! Today I kept breathing" or as complex as you want, depending on your emotional place. As children, we often heard, "Good for you!" as we completed tasks. It's time to start applauding ourselves and reminding ourselves how much we really accomplish. If you're having a difficult day, read all the things you have done. Give yourself a sticker for being you. Know that you are learning to be fully alive with grief.

Acceptance?

I use the question mark because acceptance can be complicated. People sometimes talk about acceptance as though it is a
simple thing. You magically get to a stage called acceptance, and
then everything is supposed to flow smoothly. First, there is the
question of how we define acceptance. Then there is the simple fact that when someone central to our life dies, it is normal to
accept it on one level while at the same time refusing to accept
it at all. Acceptance can be a place of peace; it can also be a
sharp-toothed alligator you never stop wrestling with.

Day One

> "You think you've accepted that someone is out of your
> life, that you've grieved and it's over, and then bam.
> One little thing, and you feel like you've lost that per-
> son all over again."

—RACHEL HAWKINS

I've given up trying to accept that my husband is dead. I'm not delusional. I
know he's dead. It's just that I keep being surprised by the recurring longing to share something with him, to see his smile, to touch his hand. I don't
think I will ever accept his death completely. There is always a part of me
that finds and loses him over and over again.

Day Two

"I discover that grief means living with someone who is not there."

—JEANETTE WINTERSON

It's what we do. We live with someone who is not there. We know they are not there. We accept their absence, but this does not stop the way we continue to have a relationship with them.

Day Three

"He did not run from his grief, nor did he deny its existence. He could study his grief from a distance, like a scientist observing animals. He embraced it, accepted it, acknowledged that it would never go away. It was as much a part of him as any pleasant feeling . . . "

—BECKY CHAMBERS

Acceptance means different things to different people. For some, acceptance is a way of letting go. Grief dissolves and slips away. For others, acceptance is acknowledging that grief will always be a part of us now. We accept that we are forever changed.

Day Four

"Slowly, painfully, I let go. It was like prying my own
fingers off the edge of the cliff. And that hurt too—
particularly the falling part, and not being sure what
was at the bottom. But I did know. *Now* was what was
at the bottom. I was already there."

—ROBIN MCKINLEY

Some grievers force themselves to let go of the past. They feel that living
in the present, in the now, is more important than anything that went
before. I honor this definition of acceptance but it differs from mine. I
never intend to let go. My then enhances my now.

Day Five

"Grief would weave itself among the threads of love
and life and hope, and I was starting to believe that
what came of it all would still one day be beautiful."

—SHANNON HUFFMAN POLSON

There can come a kind of wonder in watching grief change from an
overwhelming darkness to a multicolored group of threads that winds
endlessly through each piece of the tapestry of our life. What once seemed
only ugly and agonizing can become transcendent. For me, the great
beauty in grief, what gives it light and sparkle, is love.

Day Six

"Acceptance . . . means that even when the unthinkable happens, we honor our self and our experience with dignity and kindness. Rather than turn our back on our own suffering, we treat ourselves as we would a beloved friend."

—HEATHER STANG

Without kindness and self-care, acceptance can increase rather than diminish suffering. Whatever level of acceptance we are seeking, we must consciously remember to treat ourselves as we would the most beloved person in our life.

Day Seven

"Today I want to be real, I will not hide my pain as well as my happiness. I will not care if my gloomy face or desperate words cause concern or embarrassment in others. I do not need [to] be fed with reassuring words about the beauty of life. The beauty of life resides in the full acceptance of All That Is."

—FRANCO SANTORO

This requires constant learning and relearning on my part. My definition of acceptance means being real and looking honestly at both my life and the world around it and then accepting both. The beauty of life is not some fake construct. I want to have the courage to find beauty in the acceptance of All That Is.

Becoming a Grief Whisperer

Have a large piece of construction paper and markers ready. Think of how you define acceptance. One definition is "willingness to tolerate a difficult or unpleasant situation." When I am able I want my acceptance to be grateful and full of love.

Make three columns. In the first column write "I accept . . . " In the second column write, "I am in the process of accepting . . . " In the third column write, "I will never accept . . . " Fill in the blanks with as many things as you wish. Something may appear in one, two, or all three columns.

Revisit what you have written once a month and see if anything has changed. If things have not changed, do you accept this? If they have changed, do you accept this? If the lack of change is not acceptable is there any action you can take to make it more acceptable?

Healing?

For many grievers, healing always has a question mark after it. Some people feel that time heals and they can move on with ease. Other people believe that time fails to heal. Grief lasts, as does love, until we take our own last breath. What is your own concept of healing? I am different than I was when my husband first died. I think of healing as a daily process. I will never be healed. I may be healing. Healing includes having more happy and productive moments. It also includes crying and collapsing. Healing is like acceptance; it is honoring all that is.

Day One

"I'd never known that I could feel this broken and whole at once."

—RACHEL L. SCHADE

I say that I have fallen into the black "whole" of grief. I am still broken. My pieces still have sharp edges that don't quite fit together. Yet I am still whole. What patches my shattered self is gratitude for the love I have been given. My empty space is full of both my loved one's absence and their presence.

Day Two

"I was tired of well-meaning folks, telling me it was time I got over being heartbroke. When somebody tells you that, a little bell ought to ding in your mind. Some people don't know grief from garlic grits. There's some things a body ain't meant to get over."

—MICHAEL LEE WEST

Healing, for me, is not getting over grief. Healing is finding a home for it in my life. Healing is learning to have my grief inspire me rather than deaden me. I am not meant to get over being "heartbroke"; I am meant to learn to be fully alive while the heartbreak continues.

Day Three

"Great pain is repetitive. Grief is repetitive. And, maybe, this repetition can become a chant inside a healing ceremony."

—SHERMAN ALEXIE

Our grief can be healing or destructive. Maybe it can be both at the same time. What if the repetitive nature of grief is a sacred chant we build healing around? Someone told me that their beloved dead had become a blessing in their heart. Grief is a healing ceremony of love.

Day Four

"A few words from me won't touch your grief, and nor should they. Tend your grief like hard ground, and wait. One day, something will grow; there won't be an answer, but you will see you've found a way to live, and to live with death."

—ROBYN CADWALLADER

Have you ever seen flowers growing through a crack in a city sidewalk? Have you seen plants blossom in a desert landscape? Take actions to tend your grief and nourish yourself. You will be surprised what is still capable of growing within you. What was impossible becomes possible.

Day Five

"She remembered him smiling, and realized that time, that great old healer, had finally accomplished its work, and now . . . one was left feeling simply grateful. For how unimaginably empty the past would be without him to remember."

—ROSAMUNDE PILCHER

I cannot, do not want to even consider having had a life without my husband nor the many other people I love who have died. Healing is taking back the memories from the claws of grief. Instead of agony and bitterness, there is joy and gratitude.

Day Six

"Even as you grieve, allow light to seep through the cracks, uplift, and illuminate a healing. Baby turtles emerge from the cracking of shells; new life can burst forth."

—LAURA STALEY

Grief can build a hard shell around us. Some of us never even try to break through. We are frightened to be in the world alone. If you can hold both the dark and the light, if you can work to come out into your life once more, the healing that happens allows you to honor yourself and the life of those you love. If a baby turtle can take the risk of entering an unfamiliar world, so can we.

Day Seven

"When we lose someone we love, we can either die with them or live on to celebrate their life. I'm tired of focusing on what we lost. I want to focus on what we had."

—BARBARA DELINSKY

The most important moment in my life of grief was when I realized that I wanted my husband's life to matter more than his death. I realized thinking of him only as a dead body was disrespectful to both of us. He worked so hard in his life to overcome hardship and become a loving man who helped people. We loved deeply and laughed often. I want to make every day a celebration of who he was and what we had. Some days the loneliness still hits hard. Yet, more often now, I am thinking of him with a smile and a warm heart. For me, healing isn't letting go. Healing is holding on with love and gratitude, moving forward with love.

Becoming a Grief Whisperer

Find a comfortable space to relax into a meditation. If you wish, play soothing music or soft nature sounds. You will be creating your own imaginary healing spa. What is the setting? Is it indoors or outdoors? Is there a swimming pool, a sauna, a theater, a mirrored ballroom? It can contain anything you wish. Who works there? Perhaps the staff is all people you love who have died, or celebrities or historical figures. They can be animal spirits or other kinds of spirit guides, or holy men and women. Take it further. What is on the spa menu? It can be massages, exercise, acupuncture, or swimming, or more unusual things like magic, movies, or live storytellers.

What activities do you prefer? Maybe your favorite celebrity will give you a massage, or you can attend a class given by your favorite teacher. Perhaps you want painting sessions with da Vinci or Jackson Pollock, or to be led on a spiritual journey? If you so desire, visit with loved ones who have died. Your experiences in your healing spa are unlimited and given freely and with love. They can remain the same or change over time. When you have finished the treatments you have chosen for this moment, on this day, remember to bring the good feelings back with you into your conscious life. If you need a touch-up during a stressful moment, close your eyes for just a second. Bring whatever it is you need back to you. Open your eyes. No one will know you have been away.

EPILOGUE

My husband died at home. Because his appearance was always important to him, I tried to dress him in a silk shirt with a tie. Even with a caregiver helping me, this was an impossible task. I found his T-shirt that said, "I do all my own stunts," and that is what he wore when he was taken off into the night.

When someone you love dies, you are left to do all your own stunts. Where once you had love and support, now you have absence and longing. Grief work is finding the ways in which love and support still exist. Eternal missing is eternal love.

I hope that Grief Day By Day has been helpful in some way. We are grief warriors together. I don't like doing all my own stunts, but I am getting more adept at them. I hope someday there will be a big party in the sky that I can join in. Until that day comes, I will try to be true to myself and true to my husband.

I wish you the courage and love you need as you discover those things you wish for yourself in order to begin to feel that you are fully alive with grief.

With love,
Jan

RESOURCES

Books

Angel Catcher: A Journal of Loss and Remembrance by Kathy Eldon, Amy Eldon Turteltaub

Bearing the Unbearable: Love, Loss, and the Heartbreaking Path of Grief by Dr. Joanne Cacciatore

Comfort for Grieving Hearts: Hope and Encouragement in Times of Loss by Gary Roe

Grief Diaries (a series of books) by Lynda Cheldelin Fell

A Grief Observed by C.S. Lewis

Healing Your Grieving Heart (a series of books) by Alan D. Wolfelt, Ph.D.

I Miss You: A First Look At Death (for children) by Pat Thomas

It's OK That You're Not OK: Meeting Grief and Loss in a Culture That Doesn't Understand by Megan Devine

Living With Grief: 36 Lessons From Life edited by David Pierce and other authors (anthology)

On Grief and Grieving: Finding the Meaning of Grief Through the Five Stages of Loss by Elisabeth Kübler-Ross and David Kessler

Websites

To join Jan's Facebook community of over 2 million followers, visit facebook.com/GriefSpeaksOut.

Jan's blog, "Stop Thief: Don't Steal My Grief," can be found at GriefSpeaksOut.net.

Additional grief websites you may find helpful include:

CenterForLoss.com

ChildrenGrieve.org

Gratefulness.org/light-a-candle

Grief.com

GriefShare.org

MastersInCounseling.org/loss-grief-bereavement.html

MISSFoundation.org

PetLossHelp.org

SayingGoodbye.org

INDEX

ABOUT THE AUTHOR

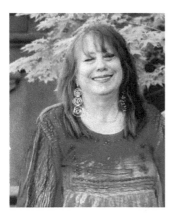

JAN WARNER likes exploring all aspects of her creativity. She has a master's degree in counseling and has worked in child abuse prevention and suicide prevention. She owned a bookstore called The Turning Page. She produced a conference called "The Resilience of the Human Spirit." The presenters were poets who have survived genocide and political terror. This was made into a Katja Esson documentary, *Poetry of Resilience*. Jan also produced documentaries, including Ferne Pearlstein's *The Last Laugh*. She produced an off-Broadway play with Hayley Mills called *Party Face*. She has also published two essays, one poem, and one short story. This is her first book. Jan loves theater, and after her husband died, she did storytelling and wrote and performed a one-woman show. Looking for renewed meaning in her life, she started a blog called "Stop Thief: Don't Steal My Grief," thinking that helping one person would be enough. Today, her Facebook page, Grief Speaks Out, has over 2 million likes from almost every country in the world. She has been to all seven continents. With all these accomplishments, the most valued part of Jan's life is time spent with her daughter Erin and her granddaughter Gwendolyn.

ABOUT THE FOREWORD AUTHOR

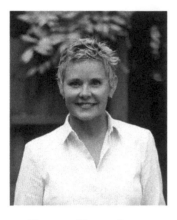

AMANDA BEARSE has enjoyed over thirty-five years in the entertainment industry. She studied acting at The Neighborhood Playhouse in New York city under Sanford Meisner, and eventually moved to Los Angeles, where she was cast in the cult horror film *Fright Night* opposite Chris Sarandon and Roddy McDowall. Following that, Bearse was cast in another cult classic, in the role of Marcy D'Arcy on the Fox sitcom *Married . . . with Children.*

Bearse directed numerous episodes of *Married . . . with Children* and she remains behind the camera as a director and producer. She co-executive produced and directed *The Big Gay Sketch Show* for LOGO, the first cable network aimed primarily toward LGBT viewers. In 2018, Bearse made her off-Broadway directing debut with *Party Face*, produced by Jan Warner.

Now living in the Pacific Northwest, Bearse is the Concentration Lead for the BA Completion in Acting Program at the Seattle Film Institute.

CPSIA information can be obtained
at www.ICGtesting.com
Printed in the USA
JSHW020911121221
21149JS00004B/4

9 781641 521314